MILADY®

STANDARD BARBERING
STUDENT WORKBOOK

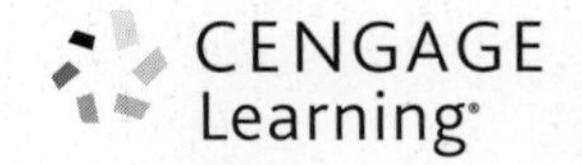

Australia • Brazil • Mexico • Singapore • United Kingdom • United States

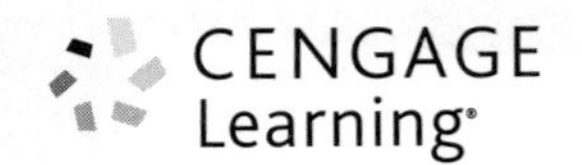

Milady Standard Barbering
Student Workbook, 6th Edition

Executive Director, Milady: Sandra Bruce

Product Director: Corina Santoro

Content Developer: Sarah Prediletto

Associate Learning Design Author: Harry Garrott

Product Assistant: Michelle Whitehead

Senior Director, Sales & Marketing: Gerard McAvey

Marketing Manager: Elizabeth Bushey

Senior Director, Production: Wendy Troeger

Director, Production: Andrew Crouth

Senior Content Project Manager: Nina Tucciarelli

Senior Art Director: Benj Gleeksman

Cover Images:
Hair: Fern Andong and Jes Sutton
Makeup: Amy Elizabeth
Photography: Joseph and Yuki Paradiso

Library of Congress Control Number: 2016934303

ISBN: 978-1-305-10066-4

Milady
20 Channel Center Street
Boston, MA 02210
USA

Cengage Learning is a leading provider of customized learning solutions with employees residing in nearly 40 different countries and sales in more than 125 countries around the world. Find your local representative at **www.cengage.com.**

Cengage Learning products are represented in Canada by Nelson Education, Ltd.

For your lifelong learning solutions, visit **milady.cengage.com.**

Purchase any of our products at your local college store or at our preferred online store **www.cengagebrain.com.**

Visit our corporate website at **cengage.com.**

Printed in the United States of America
Print Number: 06 Print Year: 2019

6 GENERAL ANATOMY AND PHYSIOLOGY | 50

7 BASICS OF CHEMISTRY | 61

8 BASICS OF ELECTRICITY | 73

9 THE SKIN—STRUCTURE, DISORDERS, AND DISEASES | 81

10 PROPERTIES AND DISORDERS OF THE HAIR AND SCALP | 92

11 TREATMENT OF THE HAIR AND SCALP | 103

12 MEN'S FACIAL MASSAGE AND TREATMENTS | 111

13 SHAVING AND FACIAL-HAIR DESIGN | 131

14 MEN'S HAIRCUTTING AND STYLING | 140

15 MEN'S HAIR REPLACEMENT | 157

16 WOMEN'S HAIRCUTTING AND STYLING | 167

17 CHEMICAL TEXTURE SERVICES | 177

18 HAIRCOLORING AND LIGHTENING | 188

Milady Standard Barbering Student Workbook strengthens your understanding of barbering by reinforcing material covered in the textbook. Complete each workbook chapter as the textbook chapter is covered in class and you will be one step closer to preparing for your licensure exam and obtaining your license!

This edition was expanded to include a wider variety of activities to engage you and to help you retain the information in each chapter. This workbook contains fill-in-the-blank, true or false, multiple choice, essay, short answer, labeling, case study, word search, mind mapping, matching, word scramble, and crossword puzzle activities. Some of these activity types will be familiar to you or are self-explanatory; however, directions for the more complicated are given below.

Case Study

The Case Study activity requires you to apply what you have learned to a hypothetical real world situation, and often asks you to describe a solution or process that you would recommend for the case at hand. Case Studies are answered in writing and are longer than Short Answers but typically less formal than Essays.

Crossword Puzzle

For Crossword Puzzles, you will first fill in missing words from the clues provided, and then use those words to complete the puzzle itself. Beginning at the number on the puzzle that corresponds to the word, write each word one letter per box – if two intersecting words don't work together, at least one of them must be incorrect!

Essay

Essay activities require written answers that are longer and present a complete thought. Essays typically have an introduction, a body with evidence that supports claims made in the introduction, and a conclusion.

Labeling

The Labeling activity will present you with a diagram or image from your textbook with the labels for specific elements removed, and expects you to fill in the missing names of the components. Terms should be written at the ends of the lines provided, so that they connect to the part they correspond to.

Mind Mapping

Mind Mapping is a method you can use to create a visual representation of a concept or group of connected ideas. Some basic guidelines for mind mapping a topic are:

- Write the main topic or problem in the center of a piece of paper. Mind Mapping activities in this workbook will have done this first step for you.
- Think about the topic and allow your ideas to flow.
- Write down key words or ideas that come to mind.
- Use lines to connect the key words to the main topic.
- Expand on the key words by creating new connections to additional thoughts or information.
- Use colors and/or symbols to highlight important information.

For an example of mind mapping, see Figure 2-10 in your textbook.

LEARNING OBJECTIVES

After completing this chapter, you will be able to:

LO1 **Discuss the evolution of barbering and the origin of the word *barber*.**

LO2 **Describe the practices of the barber-surgeons and the meaning behind the barber pole.**

LO3 **Identify the organizations responsible for advancing the barbering profession and explain the function of state barber boards.**

LO4 **Recognize the resurgence of barbering in the twenty-first century and the wealth of opportunities available to the new barber.**

Introduction

Fill-in-the-Blank

In the space(s) provided, write the word(s) that correctly complete(s) each statement.

1 Barbering is one of the oldest ________________ in the world.

2 Almost all cultures practiced some form of ________________ and ________________, given the archeological evidence found in ________________, early sculptures, and ________________.

Why Study the History of Barbering?

Fill-in-the-Blank

3 Knowing the history of your profession can help you ________________ and understand upcoming ________________.

Understand the History of Barbering

LO1 **Discuss the evolution of barbering and the origin of the word *barber*.**

Fill-in-the-Blank

4 Barbering has a rich ________________, stretching back millennia.

Ancient Cultures

Multiple Choice/Fill-in-the-Blank

5 ______________________ or strips of hide were used as adornment, and braiding techniques were employed in many cultures.

- **a.** Animal sinew
- **b.** Animal muscle
- **c.** Cow hides
- **d.** Animal products

6 Archeologists can trace the barbering profession as far back as:

- **a.** the Industrial Revolution.
- **b.** the Middle Ages.
- **c.** the Glacial Age.
- **d.** the Renaissance period.

7 What type of systems elevated tribal barbers to positions of importance, becoming medicine men, shamans, or priests?

- **a.** Belief.
- **b.** Religious.
- **c.** Value.
- **d.** Moral.

8 Many primitive cultures maintained a connection between what three things?

- **a.** ______________________
- **b.** ______________________
- **c.** ______________________

9 Which ancient civilization is credited with being the first to cultivate hair and beauty in a fashionable way?

- **a.** The Romans.
- **b.** The Egyptians.
- **c.** The Greeks.
- **d.** The Masai warriors.

10 What Egyptian barber has a statue in his honor?

- **a.** Moses.
- **b.** Ticinius Mena.
- **c.** Alexander the Great.
- **d.** Meryma'at.

11 Greek-Sicilian barbers from Sicily introduced ______________________ to Rome between ______________________ and ______________________.

12 *Barba* is the Latin word for ______________________.

13 What word comes from the Latin *tondere*, meaning "to shear"?

- **a.** Queue.
- **b.** Tonsorial.
- **c.** Anno domini.
- **d.** Henna.

Customs and Traditions

Fill-in-the-Blank/Matching

14 According to the Greek philosopher and mathematician _______________, the hair was the brain's inspiration.

15 Match the description with the term.

_____	Leader of the Macedonian troops	**a. Pythagoras**
_____	Accidentally burned his head with a torch	**b. Tonsure**
_____	1972 was the year the Roman-Catholic church abolished this practice	**c. Emperor Hadrian**
_____	Grew his beard to hide the scars on his chin	**d. Alexander the Great**
_____	Believed cutting hair decreased intellectual capacity	**e. Francis I of France**

16 During the nineteenth century in France, men and women showed appreciation for antiquity by wearing variations of the _______________, the style of the early Roman emperors.

The Beard and Shaving

Multiple Choice/Matching/Fill-in-the-Blank

17 Flint-bladed razors found in Egyptian pyramids were used by the ruling class for:

a. skinning animals.

b. shaving the head and face.

c. sacrificing slaves.

d. weapons in battle.

18 A form of tweezers was in use by the year:

a. 40,000–10,000 BC.

b. 8000–5000 BC.

c. 4000 BC.

d. 7000 BC.

19 Match the description with the term.

_____	Shaved with obsidian blades	**a. Sumerians**
_____	Clean shaven by 2800 BC	**b. Greek men of 1000 BC**
_____	Frequented local barber for services	**c. Mesopotamians**

20 In _______________, a young man's 22nd birthday constituted a rite of passage from boyhood to manhood. On this day he received his first _______________.

Trace the Rise of the Barber-Surgeons

LO 2 **Describe the practices of the barber-surgeons and the meaning behind the barber pole.**

Matching

21 Match the description with the term or years.

_____ Considered the father of modern surgery	**a. Barber-surgeons**
_____ Year barber-surgeons formed their first organization in France	**b. Paris, France**
	c. 1096 AD
_____ Most learned and educated people at the time	**d. Monks and priests**
_____ Period in which wigs became very fashionable	**e. Ambroise Paré**
_____ Duties previously performed by clergy	**f. 1163**
_____ Location of the school of St. Cosmos and St Domain	**g. 1700s–1800s**
_____ Name associated with barbers for over a thousand years	**h. 1745**
	i. Bloodletting
_____ City where The Guild of Company of Barbers-Surgeons was formed	**j. London, England**
_____ Year that barbers and surgeons were separated in England	
_____ Year barbers took over the duties previously performed by the clergy	

The Barber Pole

Fill-in-the-Blank

22 The symbolic history of the barber pole can be directly related to the technical procedure of ____________________ performed by ____________________.

23 The bottom end-cap of modern barber poles represents the ____________________ that was used as a vessel to catch the blood during ____________________.

Understand Modern Barbering's Organizations and State Boards

LO 3 **Identify the organizations responsible for advancing the barbering profession and explain the function of state barber boards.**

Multiple Choice/Matching

24 During what years did the profession's structure change and begin to follow new directions?

a. The late 1800s.

b. 1887.

c. 1929.

d. All answers are correct.

25 Match the description with the term or year.

_____ Employee groups

_____ Employer groups

_____ Year and location of the formation of the Journeymen Barbers' International Union of America

_____ Year and location associated with the opening of America's first barber school

_____ Year the first Moler manual of barbering was first published

_____ First state to pass barber licensing laws

_____ Year and location the Associated Master Barbers of America was formed

_____ Group the AMBBA represented

_____ Standardized the operation of barber schools

_____ Standardized and upgraded barber training

_____ National Association of State Board of Barber examiners

_____ Adopted barber code of ethics

a. National Educational Council

b. National Association of Barber Schools

c. AMBBA

d. Journeymen barbers

e. Alabama

f. 1893, Chicago, Illinois

g. Master barbers

h. Organized in St. Paul, Minnesota

i. 1924, Chicago, Illinois

j. 1893

k. 1887, New York

l. Shop and salon owners

m. Minnesota

Consider the State of Barbering Today

LO 4 **Recognize the resurgence of barbering in the twenty-first century and the wealth of opportunities available to the new barber.**

Essay

26 Throughout history, the trend of wearing a beard or being clean shaven was often put in place by a ruler or religious decree. In your own words, describe some of the factors that may influence a present-day gentleman, to decide to wear a beard or not? (Many of us are influenced by musicians, celebrities, athletes, and our peers.)

____

____

____

____

____

____

____

____

27 How can we as barbers keep up to date with the demands of fashion to best meet our client's needs?

Word Review

Word Search

After determining the correct term from the definitions provided, locate the terms in the word search.

______________	Latin for beard.
______________	Wrote the first barbering textbook; opened the first barber school in Chicago in 1893.
______________	A shaved patch on the head.
______________	Early practitioners who cut hair, shaved, and performed bloodletting and dentistry.

__________________ Barber employee unions.

__________________ Barber employer unions.

__________________ Associated Master Barbers and Beauticians of America.

__________________ Related to the cutting, clipping, or trimming of hair with shears or a razor.

__________________ Egyptian barber commemorated with a statue.

__________________ Most often a red, white, and blue striped pole that is the iconic symbol of the barbering profession.

__________________ National Association of Barber Boards of America.

__________________ Sicilian credited with bringing barbering and shaving to Rome in 296 BC.

P L E B S A R O R M B N E B R E M E N T S A

Y R R M S B A R A B O O R R B U O E U I O O

E M N B T R B I S A B M B T A S M A B C B N

C A A O S T E G S S P U A B A M S P S I S E

M P S S O R S E E B R M R S C S R B U N E R

I A A J T M S R B E N B B N R E R T O I U E

O A M J R E M N M A R U R B A I O E A U A A

R S M A U R R U A A I A S E G R G R M S A L

T R E B O Y R B S T B O E E E R B E E M A G

S S B A B M R A A E A E A E U E T L S E A B

E N P M N A A S T R R M R S G R O R B N L B

E N B Y B A R R R R B U R N A T B U B A E M

O U T A R T B B N A S E N T E O B O I L R E

J O U R N E Y M E N B A R B E R G R O U P S

M M R G E A N L O R R O E G T N O R B N U E

E N O E R R B T A L P S A R R S R P A A B C

B E R O R E O B B N E O R A N O B E G A G S

I M O S R R U G A A U R L O N B U G B L T Y

M A G R R M B E M G O A T E A I I P R A S N

B N R I M M L M U R N E M L E A L N S E I L

LEARNING OBJECTIVES

After completing this chapter, you will be able to:

LO1 List the life skills to put into action.

LO2 List the principles that contribute to personal and professional success.

LO3 Create a mission statement.

LO4 Explain long-term and short-term goals.

LO5 Discuss the most effective ways to manage time.

LO6 Demonstrate good study habits.

LO7 Define ethics.

LO8 List the characteristics of a healthy, positive attitude.

Introduction

Short Answer

1 List two reasons why studying life skills is important for a barber:

a. ______________________________

b. ______________________________

2 List the skills that can help you become successful in a barber shop:

a. ______________________________

b. ______________________________

c. ______________________________

d. ______________________________

e. ______________________________

f. ______________________________

g. ______________________________

Why Study Life Skills?

Short Answer/Multiple Choice/Fill-in-the-Blank

3 List three reasons why barbers should study and have a thorough understanding of life skills?

a. ______________________________

____

____

b. ______________________________

____

____

c. ______________________________

____

____

4 Barbers should have a thorough understanding of life skills because:

a. an employer will look for this in a resume.

b. it makes for a good conversation starter with clients.

c. it will give you the ability to deal with difficult circumstances.

d. it is a requirement for the state board exam.

5 Having good life skills builds ____________________, which help individuals achieve their goals.

Life Skills in Action

LO 1 **List the life skills to put into action.**

Short Answer

6 List the life skills that will assist in making you a well-rounded person:

1. ______________________________

2. ______________________________

3. ______________________________

4. ______________________________

5. ______________________________

6. ______________________________

7. ______________________________

8. ______________________________

9. ______________________________

10. ______________________________

11. ______________________________

Interpret the Psychology of Success

LO 2 **List the principles that contribute to personal and professional success.**

Essay Activity

7 In your own words, describe your definition of success.

____

____

____

____

____

____

____

____

____

____

Action Steps for Success

Matching/Short Answer

8 Match the following action description with the correct term:

_____ Speak with confidence, stand tall, and use proper grammar.

_____ Maintain the proper amount of sleep, and eat a healthy diet to maintain a successful life balance.

_____ Imagine already working and being successful.

_____ Practice doing what you are good at.

_____ Balance work life with personal life.

_____ Create positive affirmations.

_____ Eliminate self-criticism.

_____ Exercise good manners at all times.

_____ Be unique—it is a valuable asset.

a. Build self-esteem.

b. Visualize success.

c. Build on your strengths.

d. Be kind to yourself.

e. Stay true to yourself.

f. Practice new behaviors.

g. Keep your personal life separate from your work.

h. Keep your energy up.

i. Respect others.

9 List three bad habits that can prevent you from reaching your goals followed by their good habits that will help you reach your goals.

Bad habits	**Good habits**
1. ______________________	**1.** ______________________
2. ______________________	**2.** ______________________
3. ______________________	**3.** ______________________

Motivation and Self-Management

Case Study

10 As you enter this new profession of barbering, you will experience a variety of emotions throughout this course. The unknown is often intimidating and can prevent many people from taking risks. In your own words, describe some of the fears and concerns you felt or are still feeling about embarking on this new career. Explain how you will use specific information in this chapter to assist you in overcoming some of these inhibitions and set yourself on the path to success.

____

____

____

____

____

____

____

____

____

____

Your Creative Capability

Short Answer

11 To enhance your creativity, what are some guidelines you need to consider?

- ____
- ____
- ____
- ____

Design a Mission Statement

LO 3 **Create a mission statement.**

Short Answer

12 In the space below, create your very own mission statement, designed just for you. Take the time to express in words what represents you as a professional.

____
____
____
____
____
____

Set Goals

LO 4 **Explain long-term and short-term goals.**

Short Answer

13 List five of your career goals. Identify a time frame for each goal based on how long you think it will take you to complete it. Then categorize the goals into short term (months) and long term (years).

	Career Goal	Time Frame	Category
1.			
2.			
3.			
4.			
5.			

How Goal Setting Works

Short Answer

14 What are your short-term goals?

____
____
____
____
____
____

15 What are your long-term goals?

____

____

____

____

____

____

Demonstrate Time Management

LO 5 **Discuss the most effective ways to manage time.**

Multiple Choice

16 Examples of effective time management skills include:

- **a.** making daily, weekly, and monthly schedules.
- **b.** learning to problem solve and prioritize tasks.
- **c.** learning to say no, and not taking on more than you can handle at once.
- **d.** All answers are correct.

Employ Successful Learning Tools

LO 6 **Demonstrate good study habits.**

Multiple Choice

17 Which of the following is not an example of a good study habit?

- **a.** Arriving to class on time.
- **b.** Listening to music during class with headphones.
- **c.** Taking notes.
- **d.** Asking questions when necessary.

Repetition

Essay Activity

18 Learners retain information differently. Are you a visual or audio learner? Are you a kinesthetic learner? Consider how you best receive information and list some of the ways repetition will work for you as a barbering student.

Example: Lectures, demonstrations, hands-on practice.

Organization

Short Answer

19 So much information is given in class that it becomes very difficult to retain all of it easily. Give some examples below of methods that can help you break down or organize the information into smaller increments.

Example: note taking, highlighting.

Mnemonics

Short Answer

20 Think about the technology we have available today, such as tablets, smartphones, and computers. List three ways in which you can use such a device to help you remember a technique?

a. ____________________

b. ____________________

c. ____________________

Word Associations

Short Answer

21 The barbering terms listed below are found in the textbook. Come up with a word association for each term that will help trigger your memory as to its meaning.

a. Dermis ________________________________

b. Keloid ________________________________

c. Tonsure ________________________________

Acronyms

Short Answer

22 Acronyms are an excellent way to memorize information. Come up with some acronyms to help you study. For example: SHAPES (sensation, heat regulation, absorption, protection, excretion, sensation).

____

____

____

____

____

Songs or Rhymes

Short Answer

23 Songs can be very catchy. You can memorize the words to a song (the lyrics) by listening to the same song multiple times. Below, create a four-line song or a rhyme that relates to barbering.

____

____

____

____

____

Visual Study Skills

Short Answer

24 List two examples of visual study skills:

1. ________________________________

2. ________________________________

Mind Mapping

25 Mind mapping is an excellent way to visualize information. It can apply to almost everything. In this exercise, you will create a mind map example on opening your own barbershop. Reread your text on how to use a mind map to retain information. For this exercise, start with a center circle that represents your barbershop. Then break down what you think the many requirements of owning a barbershop are. Example: Equipment, furniture, etc.

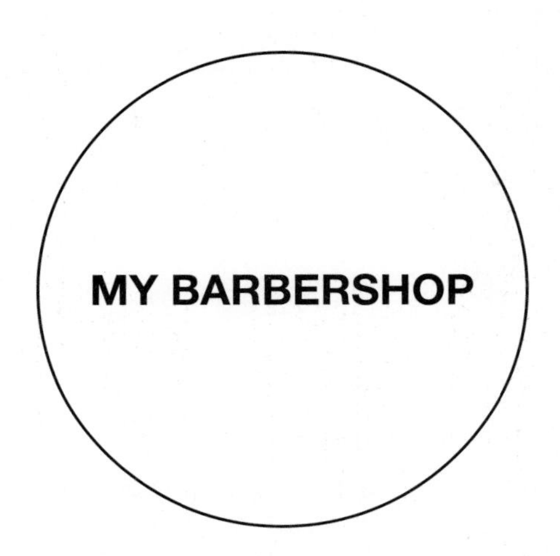

Taking Notes

Short Answer

26 Note taking is a classic way of capturing valuable information for better retention. List some tips on how to be an effective note taker.

1. ______________________________
____

2. ______________________________
____

3. ______________________________
____

4. ______________________________
____

5. ______________________________
____

6. ______________________________
____

7. ______________________________
____

8. ______________________________
____

Practice Ethical Standards

LO 7 **Define ethics.**

Fill-in-the-Blank

27 Ethics are the ____________________ by which we live and work.

Professional Ethics

Short Answer

28 Describe some qualities that an ethical person embodies:

a. ______________________________

b. ______________________________

c. ______________________________

d. ______________________________

Develop a Positive Personality and Attitude

LO 8 **List the characteristics of a healthy, positive attitude.**

Short Answer/Fill-in-the-Blank

29 List the characteristics of a healthy, positive attitude that will help every barber to interact well with all sorts of people.

1. ____________________

2. ____________________

3. ____________________

4. ____________________

5. ____________________

6. ____________________

7. ____________________

30 An individual's personality is the sum of his/her ______________, ______________, and ______________.

Word Review

Fill-in-the-Blank

Mnemonic	**Procrastination**	**Organization**
Ethics	**Goal setting**	**Perfectionism**
Repetition	**Mind mapping**	**Prioritize**
Self-actualization	**Mission statement**	

______________ The moral principles by which we live and work.

______________ Repeatedly saying, writing, or otherwise reviewing new information until it is learned.

______________ An unhealthy compulsion to do things perfectly.

______________ Putting off until tomorrow what you can do today.

______________ A statement that establishes the purpose and values for which an individual or institution lives and works by. It provides a sense of direction by defining guiding principles and clarifying goals, as well as how an organization operates.

____________________ The identification of long-term and short-term goals that helps you decide what you want out of your life.

____________________ Any memorization device that helps a person recall information.

____________________ A method used to store new information for short-term and long-term memory.

____________________ To make a list of tasks that need to be done in the order of most-to-least important.

____________________ Fulfilling one's potential.

____________________ A graphic representation of an idea or problem that helps organize one's thoughts.

CHAPTER 3 PROFESSIONAL IMAGE

LEARNING OBJECTIVES

After completing this chapter, you will be able to:

LO1 **Name four important personal hygiene habits.**

LO2 **Explain the concept of dressing for success.**

LO3 **Practice ergonomically correct movement, postures, and principles.**

LO4 **Demonstrate an understanding of human relations and communication skills.**

Introduction

Fill-in-the-Blank/Multiple Choice

1 Clients often view barbers as ______________________ experts.

2 First impressions are important in order to:

a. obtain a job interview.

b. attract new customers.

c. build a good reputation of professionalism.

d. All answers are correct.

3 List the factors that contribute to your total image:

1. ____

____

2. ____

____

3. ____

____

4. ____

____

5. ____

____

6. ____

____

Why Study Professional Image?

Short Answer

4 List four reasons why barbers should have a thorough understanding of professional image:

1. ______________________________

____

____

2. ______________________________

____

____

3. ______________________________

____

____

4. ______________________________

____

____

Apply Healthful Habits in Your Daily Routine

LO 1 **Name four important personal hygiene habits.**

Fill-in-the-Blank

5 Barbering is a profession that helps others look their best. An important part of this representation is the barber's ______________ and ______________.

Hygiene

Short Answer/Multiple Choice

6 What is one example of a basic hygiene practice?

1. ______________________________

Multiple Choice

7 What is **not** an example of good hygiene?

a. Smoking during work hours.

b. Washing your hands before and after each service.

c. Showing up to work with laundered clothes.

d. Brushing and flossing your teeth.

Rest and Relaxation

Fill-in-the-Blank/Short Answer

8 Some people need a minimum of ______________ hours of sleep to function well while others need ______________ hours.

9 Give five examples of what a barber can do while off work to help unwind:

1. ______________
2. ______________
3. ______________
4. ______________
5. ______________

Nutrition

Multiple Choice

10 Barbers need a well-balanced diet to perform at their best. Which dietary choice should be avoided?

a. Water.

b. Food containing vitamins and minerals.

c. Refined sugars.

d. Fruits and vegetables.

Exercise

Fill-in-the-Blank

11 Regular physical activity benefits the body by improving ______________, ______________, and proper ______________.

Stress Management and a Healthy Lifestyle

Short Answer/Fill-in-the-Blank

12 What is *stress*?

____

____

____

____

13 The way in which individuals perform under stressful situations depends on their ______________, ______________, and ______________.

Follow Image-Building Basics

LO 2 **Explain the concept of dressing for success.**

Multiple Choice/True or False

14 Your clients will have confidence in you as a professional if you:

a. speak highly of yourself.

b. dress in very expensive clothes.

c. present a poised and attractive image.

d. have an assistant.

15 **T** **F** You should wear cologne or perfume at all times.

Personal Grooming

Fill-in-the-Blank

16 ______________________ is the process of caring for parts of the body and ______________________ an overall polished look.

17 How you dress and how you take care of your ______________________, ______________________, and ______________________ reflects your personal grooming habits.

Dress for Success

Essay Activity/Short Answer

18 Dressing for success does not mean that you have to be someone you are not. What unique style do you possess? Do you have a modern look? Do you wish to portray a classic, old-fashioned style barber? What type of clients do you wish to attract? In the space below, *describe* how the cost of your services will determine the clothes you select for work.

____

____

____

____

____

____

____

____

____

____

19 What are some of the universal guidelines in regard to wardrobe?

a. ______________________________

____

b. ______________________________

____

c. ______________________________

____

d. ______________________________

____

e. ______________________________

____

Hair Maintenance

True or False

20 **T** **F** A barber should keep his or her own haircut and style fresh.

21 **T** **F** It is not important for a male barber to maintain his facial hair.

Skin Care and Makeup

Multiple Choice

22 Proper skin care can help to promote:

a. a professional image.
b. a big smile.
c. getting a date.
d. being pampered.

23 Applying makeup at your work station advertises:

a. professionalism.
b. good etiquette.
c. poor time management skills.
d. respect toward coworkers.

Nail Care

True or False

24 **T** **F** Manicures are a great way to relax the hands and thoroughly clean nails.

Employ Proper Ergonomics to Protect Your Body

LO 3 **Practice ergonomically correct movement, postures, and principles.**

Fill-in-the-Blank/True or False

25 Good posture conveys an image of ____________________ and can prevent ____________________ and many other physical problems.

26 **T** **F** Flip-flops are appropriate to wear in the barbershop.

Posture

Multiple Choice/Short Answer

27 Barbers may experience physical stress in all of these areas except for:

a. wrists.
b. lower back.
c. shoulders.
d. abdomen.

28 List five guidelines for maintaining a stress-free standing posture behind the chair:

1. ____________________
2. ____________________
3. ____________________
4. ____________________
5. ____________________

Body Movement

Multiple Choice/Short Answer

29 Carpal tunnel syndrome is an injury of the:

a. foot.
b. wrist.
c. arm.
d. shoulder.

30 List four suggestions on how to prevent posture problems and work more efficiently:

1. ____
____
2. ____
____
3. ____
____
4. ____
____

Practice Effective Human Relations and Communication Skills

LO 4 **Demonstrate an understanding of human relations and communication skills.**

Fill-in-the-Blank/Multiple Choice/Short Answer

31 Effective communication skills help you build ____________________ with clients and coworkers.

32 What is an example of good human relations in a barber shop?

a. Avoiding topics such as religion and politics.
b. Being punctual.
c. Being capable and efficient.
d. All answers are correct.

33 List three desirable qualities for effective client relations:

1. ____
2. ____
3. ____

Effective Communication Skills

Fill-in-the-Blank/Short Answer/Multiple Choice

34 Communication includes ____________________ skills, ____________________, ____________________, and ____________________.

35 What three steps can be used to achieve client's service expectations?

1. ____
2. ____
3. ____

36 Which of the following is not an activity that is a benefit of effective communication skills?

a. Meeting and greeting clients.

b. Imprecise haircuts.

c. Selling services and products.

d. Making contacts and networking.

Social Media

Short Answer

37 List the dos and don'ts of how to properly communicate via social media.

Do

____

____

____

____

Don't

____

____

____

____

Word Review

Matching

_____ Process of caring for parts of the body and maintaining an overall polished look.

_____ Act of successfully sharing information between two people (or groups of people) so that the information is understood.

_____ Impression you project through both your outward appearance and your conduct in the workplace.

_____ Your posture, as well as the way you walk and move.

_____ Science of designing the workplace as well as its equipment and tools to make specific body movements more comfortable, efficient, and safe.

_____ Daily maintenance and cleanliness by practicing good healthful habits.

_____ Interactions and relationships between two or more people.

a. Effective communication

b. Ergonomics

c. Human relations

d. Personal grooming

e. Personal hygiene

f. Physical presentation

g. Professional image

CHAPTER 4 INFECTION CONTROL: PRINCIPLES AND PRACTICES

LEARNING OBJECTIVES

After completing this chapter, you will be able to:

LO1 Discuss federal and state agencies that regulate the practice of barbering.

LO2 List the types and classifications of bacteria.

LO3 Define bloodborne pathogens and explain how they are transmitted.

LO4 Explain the differences between cleaning, disinfecting, and sterilizing.

LO5 Identify types of disinfectants and antiseptics appropriate for use in barbershops.

LO6 Discuss Standard Precautions and explain procedures for handling an exposure incident.

LO7 Discuss safe work practices that help prevent accidents and injuries.

LO8 List your responsibilities as a professional barber.

Introduction

Short Answer/Fill-in-the-Blank

1 List two reasons why studying infection control and safe work practices is important for a barber.

a. ______________________________

____

____

____

b. ______________________________

____

____

____

2 Since transmission can occur when using ______________________ implements, tools, or equipment, the performance of effective infection control procedures must be a top priority in the barbershop.

3 Safe work practices require that implements, tools, and equipment be used ______________________ and that you be aware of situations that can cause accidents in the barbershop.

Why Study Infection Control: Principles and Practices?

Multiple Choice/Fill-in-the-Blank

4 Barbers should have a thorough understanding of infection control: principles and practices because:

a. It will make clients look better.

b. It will make clients more comfortable.

c. It is motivating for the barber.

d. Their application is a requirement of state barber boards.

5 Barbers are responsible for employing safe work practices that help prevent accidents and injury from occurring in the ______________________.

Meet the Current Regulations for Health and Safety

LO 1 **Discuss federal and state agencies that regulate the practice of barbering.**

Fill-in-the-Blank

6 ______________________ agencies set guidelines for the manufacturing, sale, and use of equipment and chemical ingredients.

7 List three aspects state agencies regulate in the shop.

a. ____

b. ____

c. ____

8 The ______________________________ registers all types of disinfectants sold and used in the United States.

9 The ____ regulates employee exposure to potentially toxic substances and informs employees about the possible hazards of materials used in the workplace.

Understanding the Principles of Infection

LO 2 **List the types and classifications of bacteria.**

LO 3 **Define bloodborne pathogens and explain how they are transmitted.**

Bacteria

Matching

10 Match the following description with the most correct word. Choices may be used more than once.

_____ Cause syphilis, a sexually transmitted disease

_____ Cause abscesses, pustules, and boils

_____ Pus-forming bacteria arranged in curved lines that cause infections such as strep throat

_____ Cause diseases such as pneumonia

_____ Short rod-shaped bacteria that produce diseases such as tetanus and tuberculosis

_____ Spiral or corkscrew-shaped bacteria that cause Lyme disease

_____ Spherical bacteria that grow in pairs and cause diseases such as pneumonia

a. **Spirilla**

b. **Bacilli**

c. **Diplococci**

d. **Streptococci**

e. **Staphylococci**

Bloodborne Pathogens

Fill-in-the-Blank/Short Answer

11 A bloodborne pathogen is a disease-causing ______________________ that is carried in the body by blood or body fluids.

12 In your own words, explain how bloodborne pathogens can be transmitted in the barbershop.

____

____

____

____

____

____

Prevent the Spread of Disease

LO 4 **Explain the differences between cleaning, disinfecting, and sterilizing.**

LO 5 **Identify types of disinfectants and antiseptics appropriate for use in barbershops.**

Cleaning and Disinfecting

Matching

13 Match the following definitions with the most correct word or words. Choices may be used more than once.

_____	Significantly reduces pathogens on a surface	**a.**	**Sterilization**
_____	Destroys all living organisms on a surface	**b.**	**Disinfection**
_____	Destroys most bacteria and some viruses	**c.**	**Sanitation/cleaning**
_____	Second only to sterilization		
_____	Lowest level of decontamination		
_____	Process of cleaning and disinfecting a tool/surface		
_____	Requires steaming, boiling, or baking		
_____	Garbage removal		
_____	Washing with soap and water		
_____	Requires the use of chemical disinfectants		
_____	Highest level of decontamination		

Types of Disinfectants

Fill-in-the-Blank

14 ______________________ are excellent at removing grime and oils from metals.

15 ______________________ are a form of formaldehyde, have a very high pH, and can damage the skin and eyes.

16 ______________________, also known as ______________________, are very effective disinfectants that usually work in 10 minutes.

Disinfectant Safety

True or False

17 For the following statements circle T if true or F if false.

T **F** Keep the SDS on hand for the disinfectants you use.

T **F** Place disinfectants in an unmarked container, per the manufacturer's instruction.

T **F** Wear an apron and use tongs when mixing disinfectants.

T **F** Always add water to disinfectant when diluting, to prevent foaming.

T **F** Use tongs, gloves, or a draining basket to remove implements from disinfectants.

T **F** Store disinfectants in a low, easily accessed location.

T **F** Replace the disinfectant solution at least once a week.

T **F** If you get disinfectants on your skin, immediately wash the area with liquid soap and warm water.

T **F** Mixing chemicals together creates disinfectants with increased efficacy.

Infection Control Procedures in the Barbershop

Fill-in-the-Blank

18 Write the correct step number (1-13) next to each step of the *Cleaning and Disinfecting: Nonelectrical Tools and Implements* procedure:

_____ Put on safety glasses and gloves.

_____ Store dry, disinfected tools and implements in a clean, covered container until needed.

_____ Rinse away all traces of solution or soap with warm running water.

_____ Remove gloves and thoroughly wash your hands with warm running water and liquid soup. Rinse and dry hands with a clean fabric or disposable towel.

_____ Your implements are now properly cleaned and ready to be disinfected.

_____ Brush grooved items thoroughly and open hinged implements to scrub the revealed areas clean.

_____ Use a small scrubbing brush to clean implements in the cleaning or soap solution.

_____ Prepare the cleaning solution according to the manufacturer's directions.

_____ Rinse all implements with warm running water.

_____ After the required disinfection time has passed, remove tools and implements from the disinfection solution with tongs or gloved hands, rinse the tools and implements well in warm running water, and pat them dry.

_____ Immerse cleaned implements in an appropriate disinfection container holding an EPA-registered disinfectant for the required time.

_____ Remove all visible hair from your tools and implements before washing.

_____ Dry implements thoroughly with a clean or disposable towel, or allow them to air dry on a clean towel.

19 Leather is a _______________ material, and because of this a leather strop cannot be disinfected.

Common Antiseptics Used in the Barbershop

Fill-in-the-Blank

20 Antiseptics generally contain a high volume of _______________, giving them a distinct drying effect.

21 _______________ should never be used on an open cut as it destroys the cells that begin the healing process in a wound.

Follow Standard Precautions to Protect You and Your Clients

LO 6 Discuss Standard Precautions and explain procedures for handling an exposure incident.

Fill-in-the-Blank

22 Standard precautions include _______________ washing, wearing of _______________, and proper handling and _______________ of sharp instruments.

23 Fill in the blanks to complete the procedural steps that should be used when a client sustains a cut or nick in the performance of barbering services.

a. _______________ the service immediately.

b. Dispose of the blade in a(n) _______________ and place the razor in a container designated for cleaning and disinfection.

c. Face your client and calmly _______________ for the incident.

d. Excuse yourself to go _______________.

e. Once your hands are clean, immediately _______________.

f. Apply slight pressure to the area with a moistened cotton round to _______________.

g. Dispose of the used cotton round in a(n) _______________.

h. Then gently clean with a(n) _______________ and have the client wash the area if appropriate.

i. Dispose of the wipe in the _______________.

j. Dispense _______________ powder onto a cotton round and use a cotton swab to apply it to the injury to stop any residual bleeding.

k. Apply an adhesive _______________ to completely cover the wound.

l. Clean and ____________________ the workstation, as necessary.

m. Discard all single-use ____________________ objects, such as wipes or cotton balls, in a plastic bag and then place in a trash bag.

n. Thoroughly clean and completely immerse tools and implements that have come into contact with blood or other body fluids in an EPA-registered hospital disinfectant solution for ____________________.

o. Wash your hands with ____________________ and warm water before returning to the service.

Follow Safe Work Practices and Safety Precautions

LO 7 Discuss safe work practices that help prevent accidents and injuries.

Case Study

24 Avoiding Accidents and Injuries

In the barbershop, mistakes can be made and accidents can happen. It is important to take safety precautions to avoid accidents and injuries. However, if an accident or injury occurs, barbers must be professional, help clients, and prevent incidents from escalating. Imagine you accidentally burned a client's scalp with water that was too hot while attempting to wash the client's hair. How could you have prevented this accident?

____

____

____

____

____

____

____

____

____

____

25 What is appropriate attire for a barber while on the job?

____

____

____

____

____

____

____

____

26 How should you handle the challenges posed by children in the barbershop?

____

____

____

____

____

____

____

____

List Your Professional Responsibilities

LO 8 List your responsibilities as a professional barber.

Fill-in-the-Blank

27 List the responsibilities of a professional barber.

a. Never take ____________________ for cleaning and disinfecting.

b. Follow all state and federal ____________________ and rules.

c. Notify the ____________________ agency if you move or change your name.

d. Be aware of your ____________________ so that you can identify and eliminate potential hazards to make the barbershop safer for you and your clients.

e. Every shop should have employee and clientele ____________________ information available near the telephone.

Word Review

Matching

Match the following terms with their definitions.

Contamination	**Flagella**	**Tinea capitis**
Allergy	**Efficacy**	**Diplicocci**
Virus	**Immunity**	**Pathogenic**
Quaternary ammonium compound (quat)	**Nonporous**	**Microorganism**
	Bacilli	

1. ________________ Spherical bacteria that grow in pairs and cause diseases such as pneumonia.

2. ________________ An item that is made or constructed of a material that has no pores or openings and cannot absorb liquids.

3. ________________ Slender, hairlike extensions used by bacilli and spirilla for locomotion (moving about). May also be referred to as cilia.

4. ________________ A fungal infection of the scalp characterized by red papules, or spots, at the opening of the hair follicles.

5. ________________ The presence, or the reasonably anticipated presence, of blood or other potentially infectious materials on an item's surface or visible debris or residues such as dust, hair, and skin.

6. ________________ The ability of the body to destroy and resist infection. Against disease, it can be either natural or acquired and is a sign of good health.

7. ________________ Products made of quaternary ammonium cations and designed for the disinfection of nonporous surfaces. They are appropriate for use in noncritical (noninvasive) environments and are effective against most pathogens of concern in the barbershop environment.

8. ________________ A reaction due to extreme sensitivity to certain foods, chemicals, or other normally harmless substances.

9. ________________ The ability of a product to produce the intended effect. On a disinfectant label, it indicates specific pathogens destroyed or disabled when used properly.

10. ________________ A parasitic submicroscopic particle that infects and resides in cells of biological organisms. It is capable of replication only through taking over the host cell's reproductive function.

11. ____________________ Harmful microorganisms that can cause disease or infection in humans when they invade the body.

12. ____________________ Short rod-shaped bacteria. They are the most common bacteria and produce diseases such as tetanus (lockjaw), typhoid fever, tuberculosis, and diphtheria.

13. ____________________ Any organism of microscopic or submicroscopic size.

CHAPTER 5

IMPLEMENTS, TOOLS, AND EQUIPMENT

LEARNING OBJECTIVES

After completing this chapter, you will be able to:

- **LO 1** List the principal tools of the trade used in barbering.
- **LO 2** Describe when to use different combs and brushes.
- **LO 3** Discuss and identify the types of haircutting shears.
- **LO 4** Identify the parts of haircutting shears.
- **LO 5** Show how to properly hold shears for haircutting.
- **LO 6** Show how to palm the shears and comb.
- **LO 7** Describe two types of clippers.
- **LO 8** Identify the main parts of a clipper.
- **LO 9** Show different ways to hold clippers for haircutting.
- **LO 10** Name two types of straight razors.
- **LO 11** Identify the different parts of a straight razor.
- **LO 12** Show how to hold a straight razor for shaving, honing, and stropping.
- **LO 13** Show how to hold a straight razor for haircutting.
- **LO 14** Describe the functions of hones and strops.
- **LO 15** Show how to hone and strop a conventional blade straight razor.
- **LO 16** Identify the types of equipment and supplies used in barbering.
- **LO 17** Identify ways to remove hair clippings.
- **LO 18** Show how to perform two towel-wrapping methods.

Introduction

Short Answer/Fill-in-the-Blank

1 List two reasons why studying implements, tools, and equipment is important for a barber.

a. ____

____

____

____

____

b. ____

____

____

____

____

2 You should strive to purchase ____________________ items that will perform effectively and safely to get the job done.

3 When taken care of properly, ____________________ implements and tools will provide years of dependable service.

Why Study Implements, Tools, and Equipment?

Multiple Choice/Fill-in-the-Blank

4 Barbers should have a thorough understanding of implements, tools, and equipment because:

a. The barber will know when an item needs to be replaced.

b. The right items can make the barber look good.

c. It is a requirement of state barber boards.

d. They can resell them later for a good price.

5 You do not have to purchase the most expensive items, but beware of ____________________.

Learn about Implements and Tools Used in Barbering

LO 1 **List the principal tools of the trade used in barbering.**

Fill-in-the-Blank

6 As a barber, your principal tools of the trade are ____________________, ____________________, ____________________, ____________________, ____________________, and ____________________.

7 In addition, you will use ____________________ such as blowdryers and thermal styling tools to perform finishing and styling work on your clients.

Identify Different Types of Combs and Brushes

LO 2 **Describe when to use different combs and brushes.**

Know Your Comb Basics

Fill-in-the-Blank/Matching

8 The most appropriate or best comb to use ultimately depends on the ____________________ to be performed, the client's hair ____________________, and the barber's personal ____________________.

9 A(n) ____________________ is an effective choice for combing through textured or tightly curled hair.

10 Match the following applications or purposes to the correct comb style.

_____ Used for a gradual blending; has a narrow end	**a. tail comb**
_____ Used with clippers for flat-top styles	**b. wide-toothed comb**
_____ Used for general haircutting and styling	**c. flat handle comb**
_____ Used for sectioning and parting	**d. taper comb**
_____ Used on tight curl patterns	**e. pick comb**
_____ May be used for detangling	**f. all-purpose comb**

Know Your Basic Brushes

Fill-in-the-Blank

11 Styling brushes are used to control, smooth, wave, or add fullness to hair or to ____________________ the scalp.

12 A ____________________ bristle brush traps particles and polishes the hair by distributing sebum through the strands.

Know about Haircutting Shears

LO 3 **Discuss and identify the types of haircutting shears.**

LO 4 **Identify the parts of haircutting shears.**

Recognize Shear Styles

Fill-in-the-Blank

13 There are two basic styles of shears generally used by barbers: the ______________________ style with a finger rest or tang for the little finger and the ______________________ style without a tang.

14 ______________________ shears are made through a process that produces a more porous and weaker steel that does not retain its sharpness, is more brittle, and is likely to chip or break.

Know the Basic Parts of Haircutting Shears

Labeling/Multiple Choice

15 Label the parts of the shears in the following illustration.

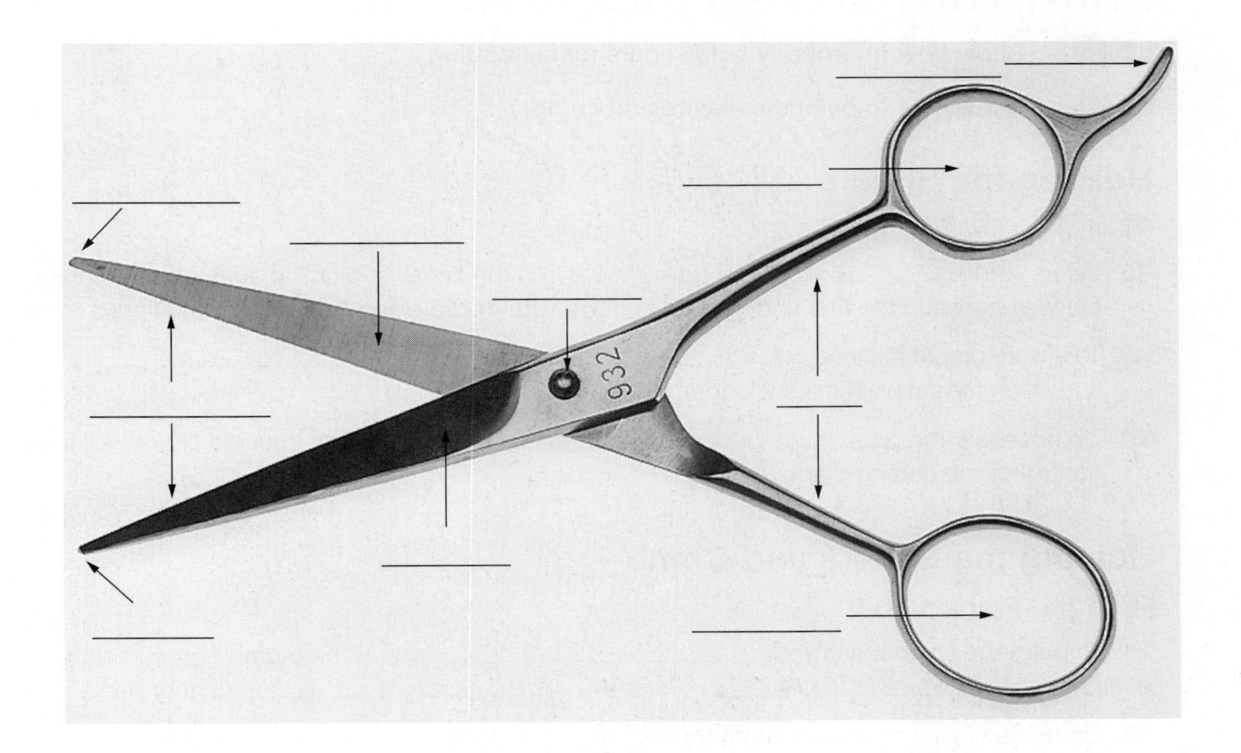

16 What handle design has a shorter thumb shank to reduce overextension and is considered to be more ergonomically correct?

a. Offset grip.

b. Heron grip.

c. Opposing grip.

d. French grip.

Describe Texturizing, Thinning, and Blending Shears

Matching

17 Match the type of shear to its description.

_____ 5 to 9 widely spaced teeth; creates patterns and texture in hair.

_____ 14 to 28 medium width teeth; differences in hair lengths are visible; adds texture and volume.

_____ 30 to 50 thin, narrowly spaced teeth that eliminate visible lines in hair; used for blending and removing bulk or weight.

a. Thinning and blending shears

b. Chunking shears

c. Texturizing shears

Show How to Hold the Shears and Comb

LO 5 **Show how to properly hold shears for haircutting.**

LO 6 **Show how to palm the shears and comb.**

Holding the Shears

Fill-in-the-Blank

18 Insert your ______________________ finger into the finger grip (still blade) approximately halfway between the first and second knuckle with the little finger resting on the finger brace.

19 To ensure proper balance, rest the ______________________ and ______________________ fingers on the shank of the still blade.

20 Do not allow the ______________________ to slide below the first knuckle or you will lose control of the cutting blade.

Holding the Shears and Comb

Fill-in-the-Blank

21 To palm the shears, slip your ______________________ out of the thumb grip and simply pivot the ______________________ into the ______________________ of your hand.

22 Once the shears have been palmed, hold the ______________________ between the thumb and first ______________________ fingers of the same hand to comb through the hair.

23 After the hair section has been combed, transfer the comb into the ______________________ of the opposite hand between the ______________________ and the base of the ______________________ finger.

Know about Clippers and Outliners

LO 7 **Describe two types of clippers.**

LO 8 **Identify the main parts of a clipper.**

Short Answer

24 In your own words, describe detachable-blade clippers.

____

____

____

____

25 In your own words, describe adjustable blade clippers.

____

____

____

____

Know the Parts of a Clipper

Labeling

26 Identify the parts of an electric clipper.

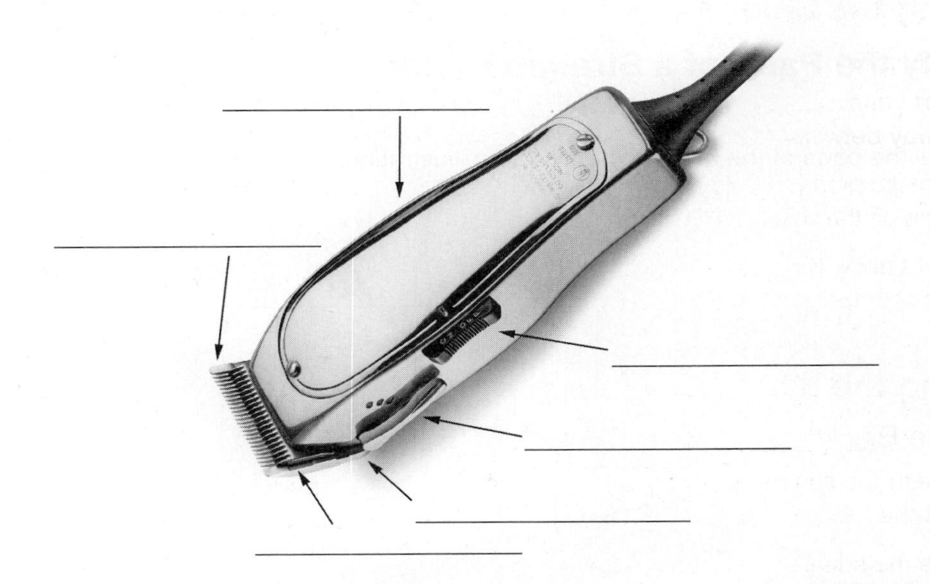

Describe Blades and Guards

Fill-in-the-Blank

27 Clipper ____________________, also known as attachment combs, are made of plastic, hard rubber, or steel for both detachable-blade and adjustable-blade clippers.

28 Clipper ____________________ are usually made of high-quality carbon steel or ceramic and are available in a variety of styles and sizes.

Show How to Hold Clippers and Trimmers

LO 9 **Show different ways to hold clippers for haircutting.**

Short Answer

29 Describe two methods for holding clippers for haircutting.

Position 1

____

____

Position 2

____

____

Know about Straight Razors

LO 10 **Name two types of straight razors.**

LO 11 **Identify the different parts of a straight razor.**

Fill-in-the-Blank

30 There are two types of straight razors: the ______________________ straight razor and the ______________________ straight razor.

Identify the Parts of a Straight Razor

Labeling

31 Label the parts of the razor in the following illustration.

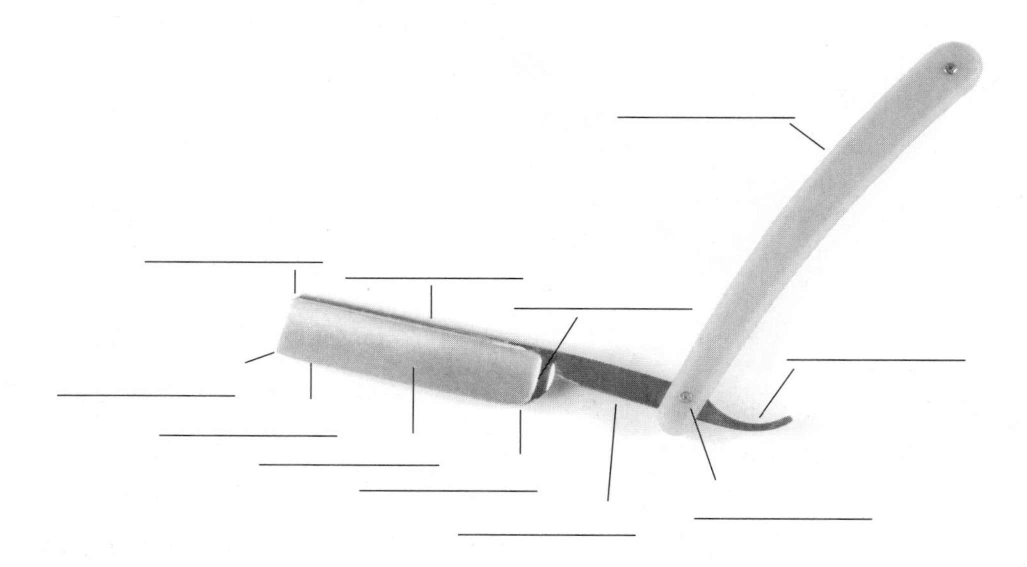

Show How to Hold a Straight Razor

LO 12 **Show how to hold a straight razor for shaving, honing, and stropping.**

LO 13 **Show how to hold a straight razor for haircutting.**

LO 14 **Describe the functions of hones and strops.**

LO 15 **Show how to hone and strop a conventional blade straight razor.**

Holding the Straight Razor

Fill-in-the-Blank

32 For shaving, the ball of the ____________________ and first two fingers are positioned on the ____________________ side of the shanks with the handle pivoted ____________________ to allow the little finger to rest on the ____________________.

33 For honing and stropping, the ball of the ____________________ and first two fingers are positioned on the ____________________ sides of the shank with the handle in a ____________________ position.

34 For haircutting, the ball of the ____________________ supports the razor at the bottom of the ____________________ and the little finger rests on the tang, with the first two or three fingers at the top of the ____________________.

Learn about Conventional Straight Razors

Fill-in-the-Blank

35 Razor ____________________ refers to the weight and length of the blade relative to that of the handle.

36 Razor ____________________ refers to the degree of hardness required for a good cutting edge, received from a special heat treatment during manufacturing.

37 The ____________________ of a razor is the shape of the blade after it has been ground. There are two general types: ____________________ and ____________________.

Hones and Strops

Matching

38 Match the following definitions with the most correct word or words.

_____ Removes any metal burrs or imbrications that remain after honing

_____ All-in-one accessory for preparing the razor after honing

_____ Produces a fine, long-lasting edge when used with water or shaving lather

_____ Produces a keen cutting edge in less time and may be used wet or dry

_____ Develops a good cutting edge and a fine finished edge

a. Natural hone

b. Synthetic hone

c. Canvas strop

d. Combination strop

e. Combination hone

Testing a Honed Blade

Multiple Choice

39 A honed blade is tested by lightly passing it over:

a. a client's cheek.

b. a strop.

c. a bar of soap.

d. a thumbnail moistened with water or lather.

40 A keen edge ______________.

a. passes over the nail smoothly without any cutting power

b. tends to dig into the nail with a smooth, steady grip

c. has large teeth that stick to the nail and produce a harsh, grating sound

d. digs into the nail with a jerky feeling

Stropping the Razor

Fill-in-the-Blank

41 The strop is attached to the ______________ of the barber chair by a closed clip.

42 When holding the razor, the ______________ finger is on the shank, the subsequent fingers are on the ______________, and the thumb rests at the pivot.

43 The direction of the blade edge in stropping is the reverse of that used in honing; therefore, the ______________ of the razor will ______________ each stroke.

44 Strokes should be made in a single, slightly ______________ stroke against the strop, with even pressure from the ______________ to the ______________ of the razor.

45 The blade edge needs to be ______________ against the surface to avoid cutting or nicking the strop.

Learn about Equipment and Supplies Used in Barbering

LO 16 **Identify the types of equipment and supplies used in barbering.**

Barber Chairs, Drapes and Capes, Towels and Linens

Fill-in-the-Blank

46 Barber chairs are larger than styling chairs, have a ______________, and are designed to enable clients to ______________ when receiving shaving and facial services.

47 The two main types of drapes used are ______________ and ______________.

48 The two types of towels generally used in the barbershop are ______________ towels and ______________ towels.

Describe the Appliances Used in Barbering Services

Case Study/Short Answer

49 Securing Appliances

Barbers must be aware of the latest and best appliances to use in the barbershop. It is important to have these items in order to provide the services clients want, to achieve the desired results, and to perform the most effectively and efficiently. Think about the services you want to provide and describe the appliances you will need to provide those services.

50 What is a high-frequency machine used for?

51 What is a galvanic machine used for?

Learn How to Remove Hair Clippings

LO 17 **Identify ways to remove hair clippings.**

LO 18 **Show how to perform two towel-wrapping methods.**

Fill-in-the-Blank

52 A ____________ or ____________ towel folded around the barber's hand may be used to remove clippings.

53 ____________ strips, may be used to remove hair clippings, although these may not facilitate a thorough dusting.

54 A ____________ system may be used to remove hair clippings, provided you clean and disinfect the ____________ attachment after each use and empty the container.

Towel Wrapping

Fill-in-the-Blank

55 Fill in the blanks to complete the procedure for performing a cloth towel wrap.

a. Grasp the towel ____________.

b. Holding your ____________ hand in front of you, draw the ____________ edge of the towel across the palm of the hand; then grasp the towel ends and twist.

c. Wrap the ____________ ends of the towel around the back of the hand and bring over the inside of the ____________.

d. Hold the ____________ of the towel while in use to prevent them from flapping in the client's face.

56 Fill in the blanks to complete the procedure for performing a paper towel wrap.

a. Grasp the towel ____________.

b. Fold down the top ____________ of the towel toward you.

c. Holding the towel at one end, insert the two ____________ fingers into the fold; maintain your grip on the towel with the thumb, ____________ finger, and fourth finger.

d. Bring the ____________ edge around the back of the hand and secure with the ____________ finger.

e. Grasp the towel end and shift to a ____________ position.

f. Wrap the remaining towel length around the ____________ of the hand and insert ____________ into the fold.

g. Continue wrapping motion around the ____________.

h. Tuck the towel end into wrap at the ____________ of the hand.

Word Review

Word Search

After determining the correct terms from the definitions provided, locate the terms in the word search.

____________________	
____________________	Plastic or hard rubber comb attachments that fit over clipper blades to minimize the amount of hair being cut with the clippers; or a metal shield applied over a haircutting razor for protection.
____________________	The technique used to hold the comb in the hand opposite of the hand that is cutting with the shears.
____________________	A comb used for cutting or trimming hair when a gradual blending from short to longer is required within the haircut.
____________________	Shears that have been made by working heated metal into a finished shape through the processes of hammering or compression.
____________________	A type of cowhide strop that is considered to be one of the best and that requires breaking in.
____________________	Usually one side of a combination strop made of linen or silk, woven into a fine or coarse texture that removes metal burrs or imbrications left after honing.
____________________	The cutting parts of the clippers, usually manufactured from high-quality carbon steel and available in a variety of styles and sizes.
____________________	Small clippers, also known as outliners and edgers, used for detail, precision design, and fine finish work after a haircut or beard trim.
____________________	A sharpening block manufactured from rock or synthetic materials and used to create a cutting edge on conventional straight razors.
____________________	Shears with 30 to 50 thin, narrowly spaced teeth that eliminate visible lines in the hair, used for blending hair ends and removing bulk or weight; also known as blending shears.

S	V	N	T	S	L	A	S	T	D	A	E	H	I
M	B	A	S	P	S	I	E	H	C	S	R	R	T
N	N	G	S	S	N	O	C	I	M	T	A	R	A
A	B	R	U	S	S	I	A	N	S	T	R	O	P
R	A	D	U	A	G	N	N	N	S	M	N	E	E
A	R	S	A	I	R	R	V	I	B	O	D	N	R
M	U	E	F	S	C	D	A	N	L	T	I	N	C
T	G	S	R	T	T	P	S	G	A	H	P	H	O
R	N	E	R	R	V	H	S	S	D	O	T	G	M
P	A	L	M	I	N	G	T	H	E	C	O	M	B
V	T	N	R	M	A	H	R	E	S	O	U	I	S
O	E	A	M	M	S	O	O	A	E	N	G	R	H
N	D	A	N	E	G	N	P	R	R	T	S	E	N
S	E	F	O	R	G	E	D	S	H	E	A	R	S

CHAPTER 6 GENERAL ANATOMY AND PHYSIOLOGY

LEARNING OBJECTIVES

After completing this chapter, you will be able to:

LO1 **Define and explain the importance of anatomy, physiology, and histology to the barbering profession.**

LO2 **Describe cells, their structure, and their reproduction.**

LO3 **Identify and define the types of tissues found in the body.**

LO4 **Define organs and body systems.**

LO5 **Name the main body systems and explain their basic functions.**

Introduction

Short Answer

1 List two reasons why studying anatomy and physiology is important for a barber.

a. ____________________

____

____

____

____

b. ____________________

____

____

____

____

Why Study General Anatomy and Physiology?

Multiple Choice

2 Barbers should have a thorough understanding of general anatomy and physiology because:

a. Clients will ask you about it.

b. Your knowledge will impress clients.

c. You will have the ability to provide appropriate services.

d. It is a requirement for the state board exam.

Why Are Anatomy and Physiology Important to You?

LO 1 **Define and explain the importance of anatomy, physiology, and histology to the barbering profession.**

Short Answer/Fill-in-the-Blank

3 Explain the importance of anatomy to the barbering profession.

____

____

____

____

____

4 Explain the importance of physiology to the barbering profession.

____

____

____

____

____

5 Explain the importance of histology to the barbering profession.

____

____

____

____

____

6 Studying anatomy and physiology builds a foundation for designing ______________ and ______________ styles or performing a proper ______________ .

7 ______________ is the study of the shape and structure of an organism's body and how body parts are organized.

8 ______________ is the study of the functions and activities of each body part.

Know about Cells

LO 2 **Describe cells, their structure, and their reproduction.**

Basic Structure of the Cell

Short Answer/Matching

9 In your own words, describe the function and structure of cells.

____

____

____

____

____

____

____

10 Match the following descriptions with the most correct structure of the cell. Word choices may be used more than once.

_____ Located in the center of the cell

_____ Encloses the protoplasm

_____ Contains less dense protoplasm

_____ Contains dense and active protoplasm

_____ Surrounds the nucleus

_____ Permits soluble substances to enter and leave the cell

a. Cell membrane

b. Nucleus

c. Cytoplasm

Cell Reproduction and Division

Short Answer

11 Cells will grow and reproduce if conditions are favorable. List three favorable conditions for cell growth and reproduction.

Favorable Conditions

1. ____

2. ____

3. ____

Identify Types of Tissues

LO 3 **Identify and define the types of tissues found in the body.**

Case Study/Matching

12 Knowledge Application

There is a lot of information to absorb when it comes to understanding parts of the body and how the body functions. This information will be useful for learning more about the barbering profession and actually providing services. Explain how you will use specific information in this chapter to assist you in providing barbering services.

____

____

____

____

____

____

____

____

____

13 Match the following definitions or functions with the most correct word or words. Word choices may be used more than once.

_____	Contracts and moves various parts of the body	**a. Connective tissue**
_____	Blood and lymph	**b. Epithelial tissue**
_____	Binds tissues together	**c. Muscular tissue**
_____	Protective covering on body surfaces	**d. Nerve tissue**
_____	Carries messages to and from the brain	
_____	Examples are bone, cartilage, ligament, tendon, and fat tissue	
_____	Controls and coordinates all body functions	

Discuss Body Systems and Associated Organs

LO 4 **Define organs and body systems.**

LO 5 **Name the main body systems and explain their basic functions.**

Fill-in-the-Blank/Short Answer

14 Organs are structures composed of specialized ______________________ designed to perform specific ______________________ in plants and animals.

15 Body systems are groups of ______________________ acting together to perform one or more ______________________.

16 Describe the functions of the main body systems.

- Circulatory: ____
____
- Digestive: ____
____
- Endocrine: ____
____
- Excretory: ____
____
- Integumentary: ____
____
- Immune: ____
____
- Muscular: ____
____
- Nervous: ____
____
- Reproductive: ____
____
- Respiratory: ____
____
- Skeletal: ____
____

Review the Skeletal System

Labeling/Fill-in-the-Blank

17 Label the bones of the cranium and the face in the following illustration.

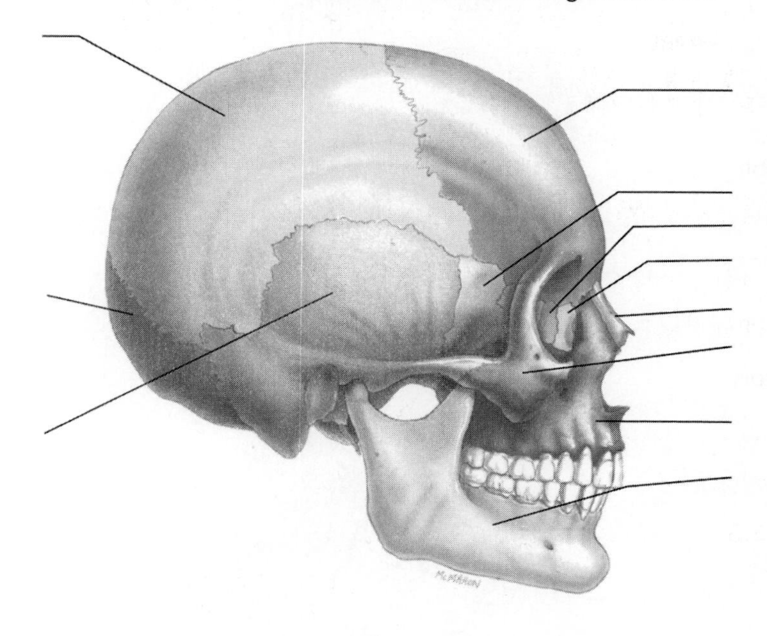

18 Painful inflammation of the carpus can be caused by ______________________ motions. ______________________ can help prevent these injuries.

Review the Muscular System

Labeling/Short Answer

19 Label the muscles of the head, face, and neck in the following illustration.

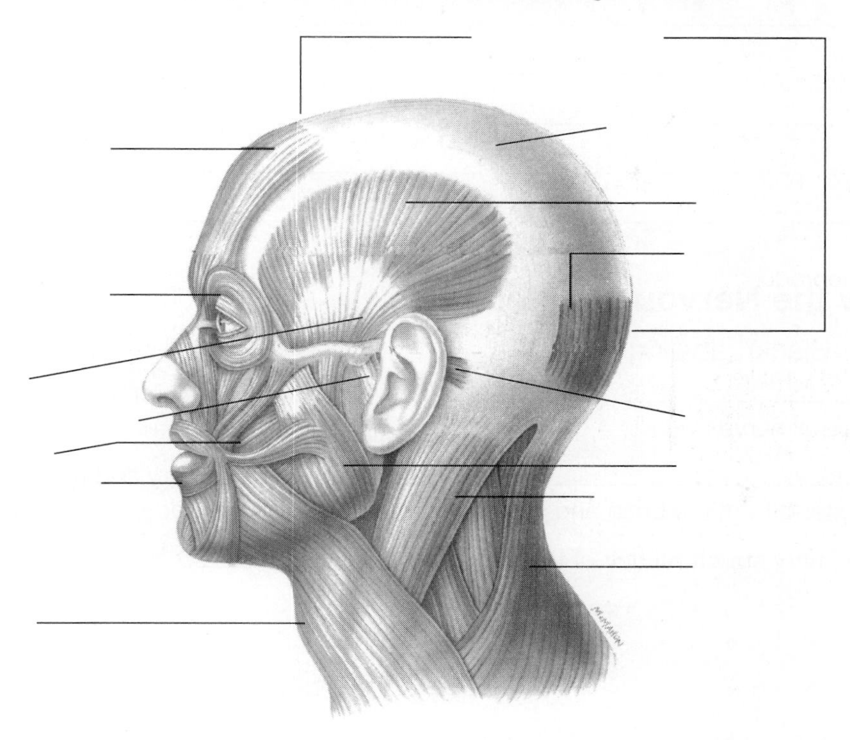

20 Label the muscles of the face in the following illustration.

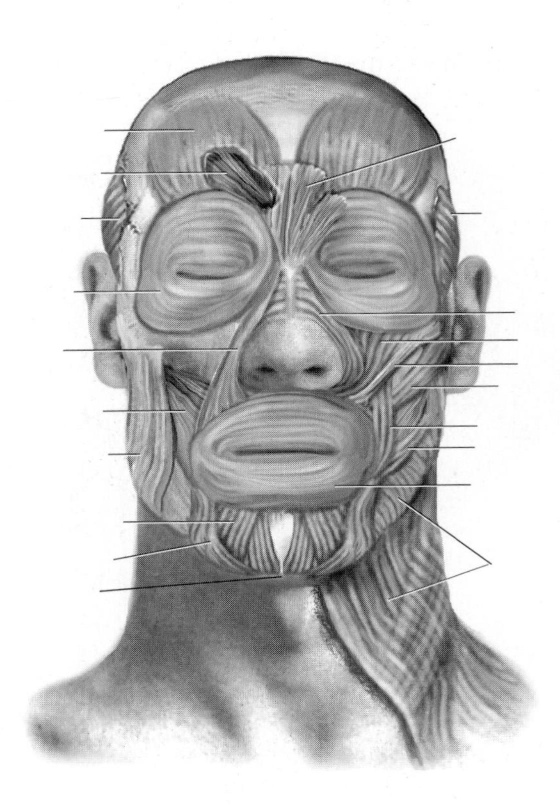

21 What methods can be used to stimulate muscular tissue?

- ____
- ____
- ____
- ____
- ____
- ____
- ____

Review the Nervous System

Fill-in-the-Blank/Labeling

22 The ____________________ consists of the brain, cranial nerves, spinal cord, and spinal nerves.

23 The ____________________ is made up of sensory and motor nerve fibers that extend from the brain and spinal cord to all parts of the body.

24 The primary structural unit of the nervous system is a ____________________.

25 Label the nerves of the head, face, and neck in the following illustration.

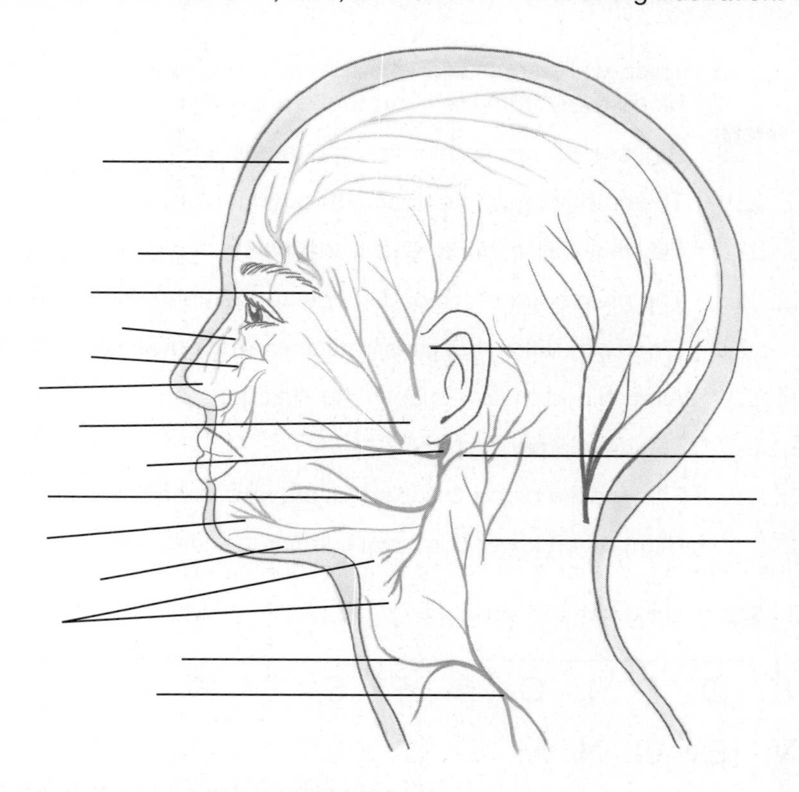

Review the Circulatory System

Labeling/Word Search

26 Label the arteries of the head, face, and neck in the following illustration.

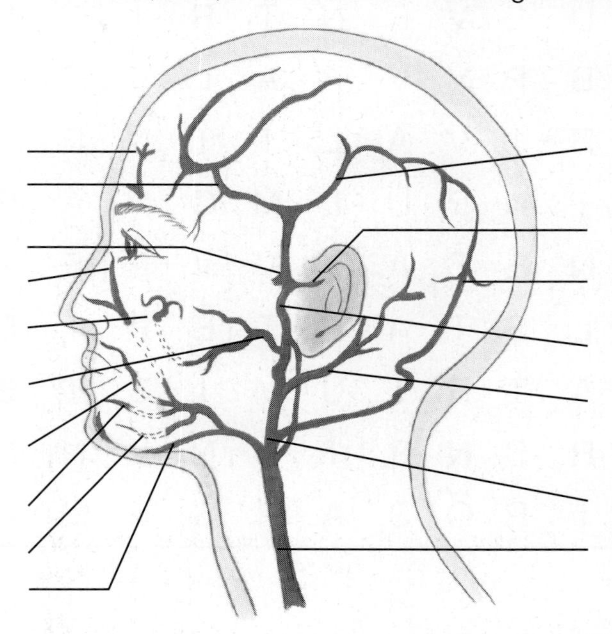

27 After determining the correct terms from the definitions provided, locate the terms in the word search.

_________________ Thick-walled muscular and flexible tubes that carry oxygenated blood away from the heart to the arterioles

_________________ Right or left upper thin-walled chamber of the heart

_________________ The nutritive fluid circulating through the circulatory system

_________________ Tiny thin-walled blood vessels that connect smaller arteries to venules

_________________ The main source of blood supply to the head, face, and neck

_________________ Blood circulation that goes from the heart to the lungs to be purified

_________________ Allow blood to flow in only one direction

_________________ The circulatory system

_________________ Thin-walled blood vessels that are less elastic than arteries

_________________ Right or left lower thick-walled chamber of the heart

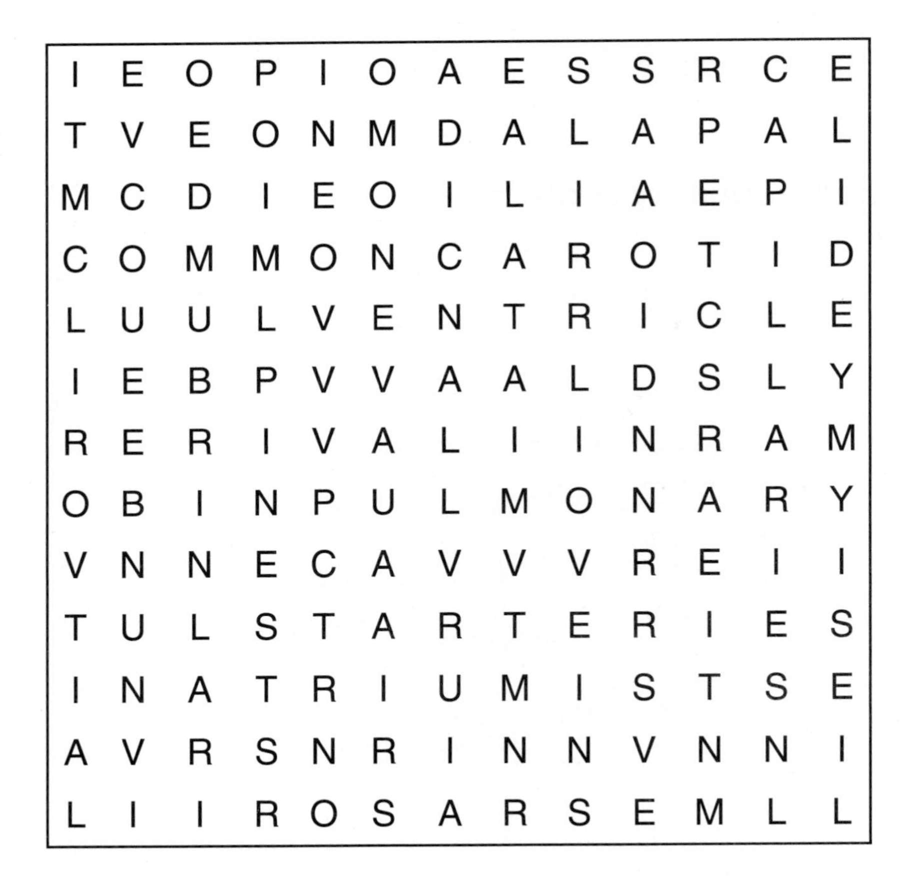

Review the Lymphatic/Immune System

Fill-in-the-Blank/Short Answer

28 The lymphatic/immune system is made up of ______________________,
______________________, the ______________________, the ______________________,
and ______________________.

29 ______________________ is blood plasma found in the spaces between tissue cells.

30 List the primary functions of the lymphatic/immune system.

- ____
  ____
- ____
  ____
- ____
  ____
- ____
  ____

Review the Integumentary System

Fill-in-the-Blank

31 Enter the correct number to complete the stats for 1 square centimeter of skin.

______________________ cells

______________________ hairs

______________________ nerve endings to record pain

______________________ pressure apparatus for the perception of tactile stimuli

______________________ sebaceous glands

______________________ sensory apparatuses for cold

______________________ sensory apparatuses for heat

______________________ sensory cells at the end of nerve fibers

______________________ sweat glands

______________________ yard of blood vessels

______________________ yards of nerves

Review the Endocrine and Reproductive Systems

Fill-in-the-Blanks/Short Answer

32 ________________________ are secretory organs that remove and release certain elements from the blood to convert them into new compounds.

33 ________________________ release hormonal secretions directly into the bloodstream.

34 ________________________ produce a substance that travels through small, tubelike ducts.

35 Four examples of hormones are: ____.

____.

36 The purpose of the reproductive system is: ________________________________

____.

Word Review

Short Answer

Fill in the definition for the following terms.

Latissimus dorsi ____

____

Risorius muscle ____

____

Bicep ____

____

Trapezius ____

____

Humerus ____

____

Metacarpals ____

____

Phalange ____

____

Centrioles ____

____

Supraorbital artery ____

____

Aorta ____

____

Endocrine gland ____

____

LEARNING OBJECTIVES

After completing this chapter, you will be able to:

LO1 Define *organic* and *inorganic* chemistry.

LO2 Define the properties of *matter*.

LO3 Discuss the physical and chemical properties of matter.

LO4 Explain oxidation-reduction reactions.

LO5 Describe emulsions, suspensions, and solutions.

LO6 Define *pH* and describe the pH scale.

LO7 Explain how product pH levels affect the hair and skin.

LO8 Name nine types of shampoos.

LO9 List four classifications of conditioners.

LO10 Recognize other cosmetic preparations used in barbering services.

Introduction

Short Answer/Fill-in-the-Blank

1 List three reasons why studying basics of chemistry is important for a barber.

1. ______________________________

____

____

2. ______________________________

____

____

3. ______________________________

____

____

2 One of the most important uses of chemicals in the barbershop is the application of ______________ and ______________ to maintain an effective infection control program.

3 List three types of products that contain chemicals:

1. ______________________________

2. ______________________________

3. ______________________________

4 Without chemicals, a ____________ change in the hair is not possible.

Why Study Basics of Chemistry?

Multiple Choice

5 Barbers should have a thorough understanding of basics of chemistry because:

a. An employer will look for this on a resume.

b. It makes a good conversation starter with clients.

c. You will be able to select the proper products.

d. It is a requirement for the state board exam.

Understand Basic Chemistry

LO 1 **Define *organic* and *inorganic* chemistry.**

LO 2 **Define the properties of *matter*.**

LO 3 **Discuss the physical and chemical properties of matter.**

LO 4 **Explain oxidation-reduction reactions.**

LO 5 **Describe emulsions, suspensions, and solutions.**

Explain the Differences between Organic and Inorganic Chemistry

Short Answer

6 Compare organic chemistry and inorganic chemistry.

____

____

____

____

____

____

____

____

Define Matter

Fill-in-the-Blank

7 Matter is anything that occupies space (volume) and has mass (weight). All matter has physical and chemical properties and exists in the form of a ______________________, ______________________, or ______________________.

8 Matter has ______________________ properties we can touch, taste, smell, or see, but not everything is matter. For example, light and electricity are forms of ______________________, not matter.

9 ______________________ are the basic building blocks of all matter and are the smallest particle that has the chemical identity of the chemical.

10 A(n) ______________________ is formed when two or more atoms combine chemically in definite (fixed) proportions.

11 A(n) ______________________ is the simplest form of chemical matter and cannot be broken down into a simpler substance without a loss of identity.

Identify the States of Matter

Labeling

12 Label the states of matter in the following illustration.

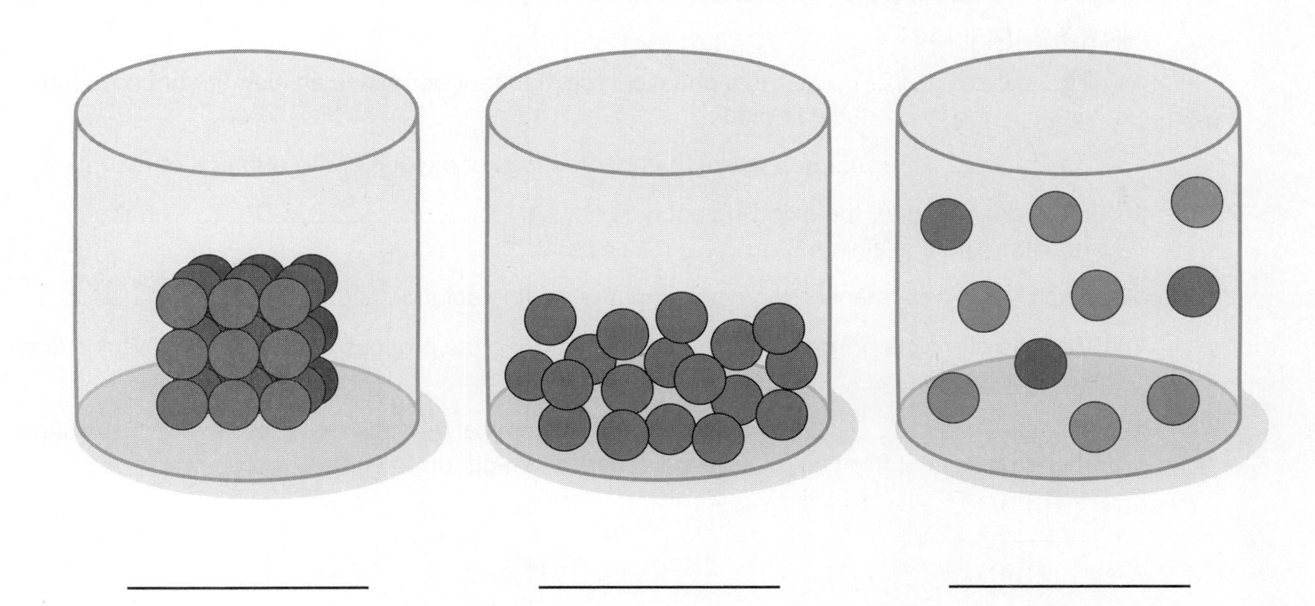

______________________ ______________________ ______________________

Understand the Physical and Chemical Properties of Matter

Fill-in-the-Blank

13 Mark the following items with a P if they represent physical properties or changes, or a C if they represent chemical properties or changes.

___ boiling point

___ burning wood

___ color

___ density

___ hair lightening

___ hardness

___ ice melting

___ odor

___ permanent haircolor

___ rusting iron

___ solubility

___ temporary haircolor

___ weight

Explain Oxidation-Reduction Reactions

Fill-in-the-Blank

14 ________________________ is a chemical reaction that combines an element or compound with oxygen to produce an oxide.

15 ________________________ refers to either the loss of oxygen or the addition of hydrogen.

16 In a redox reaction, the oxidizing agent is always ________________________ and the reducing agent is always ________________________.

17 When using a permanent wave solution, the waving solution is ________________________.

18 The loss of oxygen in the hydrogen peroxide during the process of mixing hair coloring is an example of ________________________.

19 A(n) ________________________ reaction is a chemical reaction that requires the absorption of energy or heat from an external source for the reaction to actually occur.

Identify Pure Substances, Physical Mixtures, and Chemical Compounds

Matching/Multiple Choice

20 Match the following attributes with the correct answer. Choices may be used more than once.

___	created through a reaction that changes the properties of the elements	**a. pure substances**
___	examples: oxygen, aluminum, gold	**b. physical mixtures**
___	mixed in any proportion	**c. chemical compounds**
___	examples: salt water, pure air, concrete, powders	
___	examples: water (H_20), salt (NaCl), ammonia	
___	composition does not vary	

21 ______________________ are compounds that are formed by the reaction of acids and bases.

a. Oxides

b. Acids

c. Alkalis

d. Salts

22 ______________________ are compounds of any element combined with oxygen.

a. Oxides

b. Acids

c. Alkalis

d. Salts

Define Suspensions, Solutions, and Emulsions

Fill-in-the-Blank/Matching

23 The differences between solutions, suspensions, and emulsions are determined by the types of ______________________, the ______________________ of the particles, and the ______________________ of the substances.

24 In a(n) ______________________, droplets of oil are dispersed in water, where they are surrounded by ______________________. In a(n) ______________________, droplets of water are dispersed in oil, where they are surrounded by ______________________.

25 Match the following examples with the correct answer. Choices may be used more than once.

___	witch hazel	**a. emulsion**
___	shampoo	**b. suspension**
___	calamine lotion	**c. solution**
___	mayonnaise	
___	conditioner	
___	paint	

Discuss the Properties of Water and pH

LO 6 **Define *pH* and describe the pH scale.**

LO 7 **Explain how product pH levels affect the hair and skin.**

Learn about Water and Potential Hydrogen (pH)

Fill-in-the-Blank

26 The letters pH denote ____________________, which is the relative degree of ____________________ or ____________________ of a substance.

27 The pH scale measures the concentration of ____________________ ions in acidic and alkaline water-based solutions.

28 A negatively charged ion is called a(n) ____________________, and a positively charged ion is called a ____________________.

29 A pH ____________________ 7 indicates an acidic solution, a pH of ____________________ is a neutral solution, and a pH ____________________ 7 indicates an alkaline solution.

30 A pH of 8 is ____________________ times more alkaline than a pH of 6.

31 ____________________ contract and harden the hair and tighten the skin.

32 ____________________ soften and swell the hair.

33 Fill in the effects of acids and alkalis on the hair in the table below.

Solution	Effect on Hair		Important Features
Very Strong Acid (pH 0.0—1.0)			Must not be applied to hair or scalp.
Strong to Mild Acid (pH 1.0—4.5)			Acid or cream rinses restore body to bleached, porous hair. Conditioners and fillers overcome the excess porosity of damaged hair. Special shampoos reduce tangling and matting of hair and prevent color loss. Hair creams increase sheen. Color rinses provide temporary effect. Neutralizers remove residual waving lotion.

Solution	Effect on Hair		Important Features
Neutral (pH 4.5–5.5)			Neutral solutions are designed to prevent excess swelling of normal and damaged hair. Mild shampoos for normal cleaning and manageability of hair.
Mild Alkali (pH 5.5–10.0)			Tints and bleaches penetrate easier and chemical action increases. Cold wave solutions for resistant hair. Soap shampoos to overcome acidity of tap water. Activators for hydrogen peroxide.
Stronger Alkali (pH 10.0–14.0)			Must not be applied to hair or scalp unless used as relaxers or depilatories.

Identify Cosmetic Preparations Used in Barbering

LO 8 Name nine types of shampoos.

LO 9 List four classifications of conditioners.

LO 10 Recognize other cosmetic preparations used in barbering services.

Learn about Shampoos and Conditioners

Short Answer/Fill-in-the-Blank

34 An effective shampoo product should:

- ______________________________
- ______________________________
- ______________________________
- ______________________________

35 Shampoo emulsions usually range between ______________________ and ______________________ on the pH scale.

36 Shampoos consist of two main ingredients: ______________________ and ______________________.

Identify Types of Shampoos

Matching

37 Match the shampoo characteristic with the shampoo type.

___ washes away excess oiliness without causing dryness	**a. pH-balanced**
___ cuts through product buildup	**b. balancing**
___ draws moisture into the hair	**c. clarifying**
___ rebalances and restores the pH level	**d. color-enhancing**
___ contains antifungal agents	**e. conditioning**
___ provides slight color changes	**f. medicated**
___ does not strip natural oils from the hair	**g. neutralizing**
___ usually contains citric, lactic, or phosphoric acid	**h. sulfate-free**
___ designed to clean hair systems	**i. hair replacement/wig**

Identify Types of Conditioners

Fill-in-the-Blank

38 ______________________ conditioners sometimes require longer processing time or the application of heat before being rinsed out.

39 Thermal protectors and blow-drying sprays are examples of ______________________ conditioners.

40 ______________________ conditioners usually have a lower pH than the hair, which helps close the cuticle scales.

41 ______________________ conditioners are formulated to help control minor dandruff and scalp conditions.

Review Styling Aids, Other Cosmetic Preparations, and the USP

Word Search/Short Answer

42 After determining the correct terms from the descriptions provided, locate the terms in the word search.

________________	for active correction of a scalp condition such as itching
________________	made by mixing plant oils or animal fats with strong alkaline substances
________________	protect the skin from the harmful ultraviolet rays of the sun
________________	works as an astringent and skin freshener
________________	contain humectants
________________	neutralize acids or raise the pH of hair products
________________	help the hands glide over the skin

______________ special type of oil used in hair conditioners and as water-resistant lubricant

______________ give shine and manageability to dry or curly hair

______________ stimulate scalp circulation, remove loose dandruff, etc.

______________ holds the finished style

______________ functions as a solvent in shampoos, conditioners, and many styling products

______________ remove hair by pulling it out of the follicle

______________ dissolve hair at the skin line

______________ have an alcohol content of up to 35 percent

W I T C H H A Z E L T M I A A Y G N
N S P L Z A I E I S C O I E A T O N
O W I S I L I C O N E S Y R S S A O
T P I H P N T R P T S D P Z T A A T
R S N I A E E H T I E S L N T L L C
C I D E P I L A T O R I E S L K T P
M O I S T U R I Z I N G C R E A M S
C I O N N S L D A L N I M S I N E S
N T O D W T E H R I A L C O H O L L
M A S S A G E C R E A M S S P L T R
H E E P I L A T O R S E E S I A L I
P I G S R N S G S M I S T S O M A E
C A S M N A O P E D A I I A L I S S
D G S U N T A N L O T I O N S N S S
A I A L G O A N N A I L R L G E T A
C O I H S C A L P L O T I O N S N A
D R C N A A A G L P T S T G I O G O
L R C O S O C A I G C I E P T S A I

43 Matching Products to Hair Types

It is the barber's responsibility to be knowledgeable about the products used in the shop or salon and how they can best serve the client's particular needs. Discuss the specific shampoo and conditioning products suitable for different hair types and textures: straight; wavy, curly, extremely curly; and dry and damaged hair in fine, medium and coarse textures.

Word Review

Short Answer

Fill in the correct definitions for the key terms below.

Alkali

Balancing shampoo

Clarifying shampoo

Element

Hair tonic

Instant conditioner

Liquid-dry shampoo

Molecule

Organic chemistry

pH scale

Reduction

Solution

Therapeutic medicated shampoo

LEARNING OBJECTIVES

After completing this chapter, you will be able to:

LO1 **Define *electricity*.**

LO2 **Define common electrical terms and measurements.**

LO3 **Describe electrical safety devices.**

LO4 **Examine the modalities a barber might be able to utilize depending on state licensing regulations.**

LO5 **Explain the electromagnetic spectrum, visible spectrum of light, and invisible light.**

LO6 **Identify devices used in light therapy treatments.**

Introduction

Short Answer/Fill-in-the-Blank

1 List two reasons why studying basics of electricity is important for a barber.

a. ____

____

____

____

b. ____

____

____

____

2 Different ____________________ have different effects on the skin.

3 Barbers need to know when it is appropriate to apply the thermal and chemical properties associated with ____________________ to the skin.

Why Study Basics of Electricity?

Multiple Choice

4 Barbers should have a thorough understanding of basics of electricity because:

- **a.** Clients will ask barbers to fix their hair appliances for them.
- **b.** They may need to rewire equipment.
- **c.** They need to minimize the risk of fires caused by faulty wiring.
- **d.** They will be required to read wiring diagrams.

Understand Electricity

LO 1 **Define *electricity*.**

LO 2 **Define common electrical terms and measurements.**

Fill-in-the-Blank

5 Electricity is not matter because it does not occupy ____________________ or have ____________________.

6 Electricity is a form of energy that produces ____________________, ____________________, ____________________, or ____________________ effects when in motion.

7 ____________________ is the flow of electricity along a conductor.

8 A ____________________ is any substance, material, or medium that conducts electricity.

Types of Electric Current

Fill-in-the-Blank/Matching

9 ____________________ is a rapid and interrupted current, flowing first in one direction and then in the opposite direction, that produces a ____________________ action.

10 A ____________________ is an apparatus found within a power supply or adapter that converts AC to DC.

11 Match the following description with the correct unit of measurement.

_____	Electrical resistance in an electric current	**a. Watt**
_____	Strength or rate of an electric current in a conductor	**b. Ohm**
_____	Unit of power	**c. Volt**
_____	Electrical pressure	**d. Ampere**

Practice Electrical Equipment Safety

LO 3 **Describe electrical safety devices.**

Safety Devices

Fill-in-the-Blank

12 A fuse is a safety device that prevents the ______________________ of electrical wires by preventing excessive ______________________ from passing through a circuit.

13 A fuse blows or melts when a wire becomes too ______________________, which happens when the circuit is ______________________ with too much current.

14 A circuit breaker is a ______________________ that automatically ______________________ or ______________________ an electric circuit at the first indication of an overload.

15 When wires become too hot, a circuit breaker will click off and ______________________ the ______________________.

16 All electrical appliances must have at least ______________________ electrical connections.

17 ______________________ provides protection from electrical shock in the event of a short circuit.

18 The different sizes of the ______________________ on modern electrical plugs guarantee that the plugs can only be ______________________ one way.

19 A ground fault interrupter is an outlet that senses ______________________ within an electric circuit.

Guidelines for Safe Use of Electrical Equipment

True or False

20 For the following statements circle T if true or F if false.

T	**F**	Study the instructions *before* using any electrical equipment.
T	**F**	Keep appliances connected when not in use.
T	**F**	Repair all wires, plugs, and equipment yourself.
T	**F**	Inspect all electrical equipment frequently.
T	**F**	Do not overload outlets and power strips.
T	**F**	Avoid letting electrical cords dry out.
T	**F**	When using electrical equipment, protect the client at all times.
T	**F**	Do not touch any glass while using an electrical appliance.
T	**F**	Do not handle electrical equipment with wet hands.
T	**F**	Do not allow the client to touch any rubber surfaces while being treated with electrical equipment.
T	**F**	Do not stand in the same room while a client is connected to an electrical device.
T	**F**	Do not attempt to clean around an electrical outlet while equipment is unplugged.
T	**F**	Do not touch two metallic objects at the same time if either is connected to an electric current.
T	**F**	Do not allow two electrical cords to touch while in use.
T	**F**	Do not allow electrical cords to become twisted or bent.
T	**F**	Disconnect appliances by pulling on the cord, not on the plug.

Understand Terminology Associated with Electrotherapy

LO 4 **Examine the modalities a barber might be able to utilize depending on state licensing regulations.**

Fill-in-the-Blank

21 ______________________ and ______________________ are commonly referred to as electrotherapy.

22 Different types of electric currents are used for electrotherapy, each producing a different effect on the skin. These different types of currents are called ______________________.

Define *Polarity*

Matching

23 Match the following characteristics with the type of electrode they describe.

_____ Positive **a. Cathode**

_____ Negative **b. Anode**

_____ Black

_____ Red

Explain Modalities

Case Study/Fill-in-the-Blank

24 Using Modalities

Rules and regulations for barbering vary from state to state, including what modalities barbers are allowed to work with. Determine the type of modalities that can be used in your state, and think of some possible reasons that other types of modalities may not be permitted, in your state or others.

____

____

____

____

____

____

____

____

____

____

____

____

____

____

____

____

25 ____________________ is used to facilitate deep pore cleansing. During this process ____________________ is used to create a chemical reaction that acts to emulsify sebum and waste in the pores.

26 Iontophoresis uses both ____________________ of the galvanic machine, and takes place in one of two ways: ____________________ and ____________________.

27 Identify the modalities used in the images below.

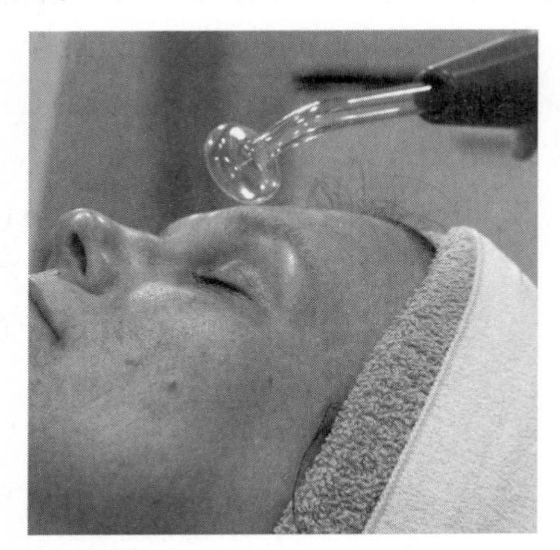

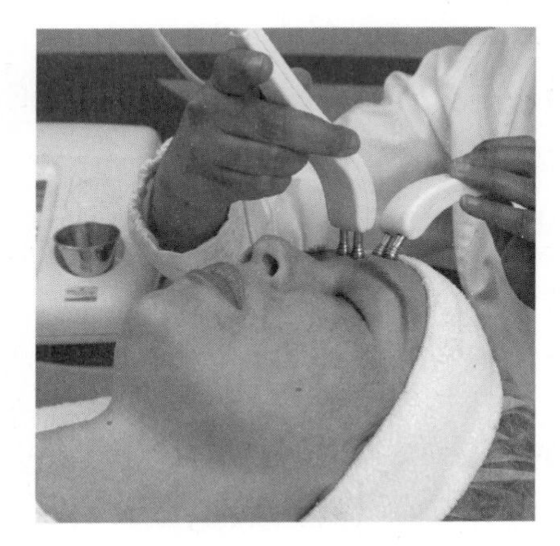

a. ______________________ **b.** ______________________

Explain Light Energy and Light Therapy

LO 5 **Explain the electromagnetic spectrum, visible spectrum of light, and invisible light.**

LO 6 **Identify devices used in light therapy treatments.**

Fill-in-the-Blank

28 The form of energy used in light therapy services are ______________________ waves.

29 Each type of energy has its own ______________________, the distance between successive peaks of electromagnetic waves.

30 Short wavelengths have a ______________________ frequency because the waves pass more frequently within a given length of time.

31 Within the visible spectrum of light, ______________________ has the shortest wavelength and ______________________ has the longest.

Visible and Invisible Light

Fill-in-the-Blank/Matching

32 Visible light makes up only ______________________ percent of natural sunlight.

33 ______________________ rays and ______________________ rays are forms of electromagnetic energy that are invisible to the human eye.

34 Match the following characteristics with the correct category of ultraviolet (UV) rays. Choices may be used more than once.

_____ The most germicidal UV rays	**a. UVA rays**
_____ Used in tanning booths	**b. UVB rays**
_____ Most penetrating UV rays	**c. UVC rays**
_____ Cause the most burning to the skin	
_____ Longest of all the UV rays	
_____ Destructive to bacteria	

Light Therapy: Lasers, Light-Emitting Diodes, and Therapeutic Lamps

35 Match the following characteristics with the correct light therapy device. Answer choices may be used more than once.

a. Laser
b. Light-emitting diode (LED)
c. Therapeutic lamp

_____ Triggers a reaction such as stimulating circulation or reducing bacteria

_____ Consists of a dome-shaped reflector mounted on a pedestal

_____ Uses blue light to reduce acne and bacteria

_____ Works by selective photothermolysis

_____ Uses red light to aid the penetration of creams into the skin

_____ Used for hair removal and various skin treatments

_____ Improves lymphatic flow, detoxifies, and increases circulation

_____ May be classified as a Level II or above medical device

Word Review

Short Answer

Fill in the definition for the following terms.

Alternating current

____

____

Cathode

____

____

Desincrustation

____

____

Electric current

____

____

Fuse

____

____

Galvanic current

Infrared light

Laser

Modalities

ohm

Polarity

Rectifier

Tesla high-frequency current

Ultraviolet light

Volt

Wavelength

CHAPTER 9

THE SKIN—STRUCTURE, DISORDERS, AND DISEASES

LEARNING OBJECTIVES

After completing this chapter, you will be able to:

LO1 **Describe the structure and divisions of the skin.**

LO2 **List the functions of the skin.**

LO3 **Identify and describe common primary and secondary skin lesions.**

LO4 **Describe common skin inflammations and infections.**

LO5 **List and describe disorders of the sebaceous and sudoriferous glands.**

LO6 **List and describe types of skin pigmentations.**

LO7 **Identify common skin hypertrophies.**

LO8 **Identify and describe types of skin cancer.**

Introduction

Short Answer/Fill-in-the-Blank

1 List the purposes of the skin.

a. ______________________________

____

b. ______________________________

____

c. ______________________________

____

2 ____________ is a branch of medical science that pertains to the study of the skin – its nature, structure, functions, diseases, and treatment.

Why Study the Skin—Structure, Disorders, and Diseases?

Short Answer

3 List three reasons why it is important to have a thorough understanding of the skin—structure, disorders, and diseases.

a. ______________________________

____

____

____

____

b. ______________________________

____

____

____

____

c. ______________________________

____

____

____

____

Know the Anatomy of the Skin

LO 1 **Describe the structure and divisions of the skin.**

LO 2 **List the functions of the skin.**

Fill-in-the-Blank

4 The skin is thinnest on the ______________ and thickest on the ______________ and ______________.

5 The skin is constructed of two clearly defined divisions: the ______________ and the ______________.

Epidermis and Dermis

Matching/Labeling/Fill-in-the-Blank

6 Review the following characteristics of the layers of the epidermis and then match the descriptions with the correct stratum or layer. Answer choices may be used more than once.

_____ Lies beneath the stratum corneum
_____ Consists of granular cells
_____ Responsible for epidermal growth
_____ Outermost epidermal layer
_____ The clear layer
_____ The spiny layer
_____ The horny layer
_____ Deepest epidermal layer
_____ The granular layer
_____ The basal cell layer
_____ Contains keratin and sebum
_____ Contains melanin
_____ Consists of transparent cells
_____ Protects against UV rays

a. Stratum corneum
b. Stratum lucidum
c. Stratum granulosum
d. Stratum germinativum
e. Stratum spinosum

7 Label the layers of the skin in the spaces below using the diagram as your guide.

a. ____________________
b. ____________________
c. ____________________
d. ____________________
e. ____________________
f. ____________________
g. ____________________
h. ____________________
i. ____________________

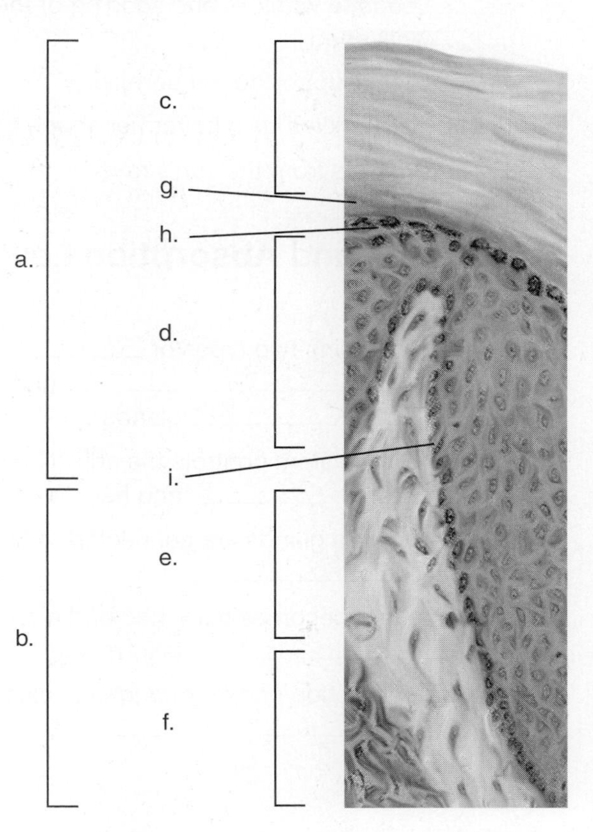

8 ______________________ tissue, also known as ______________________ tissue, is a layer of fatty tissue found below the dermis.

Fluids and Nerves of the Skin

Fill-in-the-Blank/Short Answer

9 ______________________ and ______________________ supply nourishment to the skin in the form of protein, carbohydrates, and fat.

10 Describe the function of the three classifications of nerve fibers with endings in the skin.

a. Motor nerve fibers: ____.
____

b. Sensory nerve fibers: ____
____.

c. Secretory nerve fibers: ____
____

Skin Color and Elasticity

Matching

11 Match the correct protein with the descriptions below.

_____ Gives skin color

_____ Gives skin its elasticity and flexibility

_____ Leads to wrinkles and sagging of the skin when weakened

_____ Gives support to the dermis

_____ Helps skin regain its former shape after expanding

_____ Protects from the sun's rays

a. Melanin

b. Collagen

c. Elastin

The Glands and Absorption Level of the Skin

Fill-in-the-Blank

12 The skin contains two types of ______________________ glands, the sudoriferous glands, or ______________________ glands, and the sebaceous glands, or ______________________ glands.

13 The nervous system controls the activity of sudoriferous glands, which ______________________ and help to ______________________ from the body.

14 The sebaceous glands are connected to the ______________________, where they create ______________________.

15 When sebum becomes hardened and a duct becomes blocked, a ______________________ is formed.

16 Limited absorption occurs through the skin ______________________, ______________________, ______________________, and ______________________.

Functions of the Skin

Word Search

17 Find the six functions of the skin in the word search and write them in the blanks below.

H	S	T	P	O	A	I	N	N	N	O	O	T	I
E	E	X	C	R	E	T	I	O	N	S	A	I	A
A	E	T	U	I	O	L	I	R	L	E	A	P	R
T	E	O	T	T	O	T	R	A	U	C	I	O	N
R	R	R	C	R	P	R	E	A	S	R	E	O	N
E	R	E	X	R	I	N	B	C	E	E	I	I	A
G	S	I	O	P	I	A	O	T	T	T	I	R	T
U	R	S	R	A	I	T	P	E	A	I	U	T	C
L	B	A	E	R	E	I	E	S	N	O	O	B	E
A	R	T	P	E	O	C	N	E	S	N	N	N	E
T	A	E	N	E	O	E	I	O	T	O	U	I	T
I	I	N	N	G	S	N	S	R	S	O	A	G	P
O	T	O	O	R	G	A	E	A	R	T	R	R	U
N	R	E	O	I	P	E	H	T	A	R	T	E	O

1. ____________________

2. ____________________

3. ____________________

4. ____________________

5. ____________________

6. ____________________

Identify Disorders and Diseases of the Skin

LO 3 Identify and describe common primary and secondary skin lesions.

LO 4 Describe common skin inflammations and infections.

Lesions of the Skin

Fill-in-the-Blank

18 Lesions can indicate ____________________ and may be symptomatic of other ____________________.

19 Do not perform services on ____________________, whether it is infectious or not.

Primary Lesions of the Skin

Fill-in-the-Blank

20 ____________________ lesions are often differentiated by size and layers of skin affected.

21 Identify the primary lesions in the blank column below.

Primary Lesion	Graphic	Description
	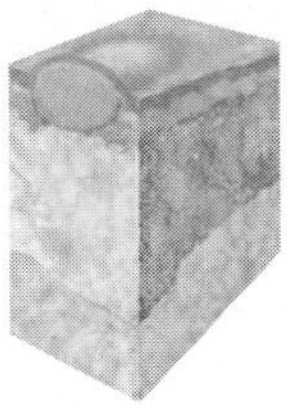	Closed, abnormally developed sac that contains pus, semifluid, or morbid matter, above or below the skin
	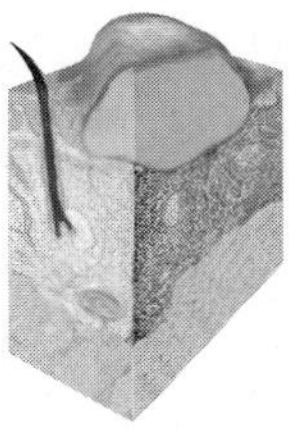	Large blister containing a watery fluid; similar to a vesicle
	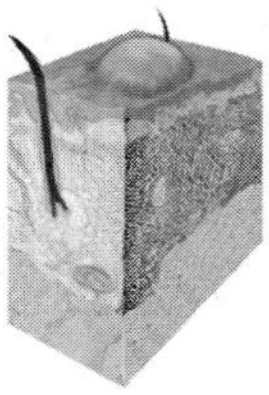	A solid bump larger than 0.4 inches (1 cm) that can be easily felt
	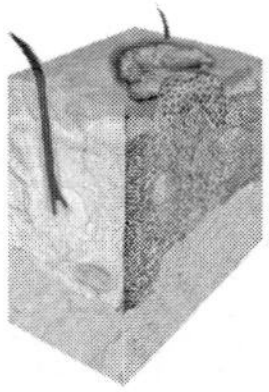	Abnormal mass varying in size, shape, and color. Any type of abnormal mass, not always cancer
	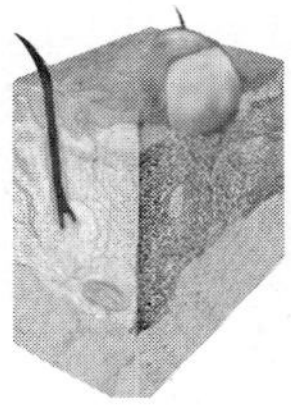	Raised, inflamed, papule with a white or yellow center containing pus in the top of the lesion
	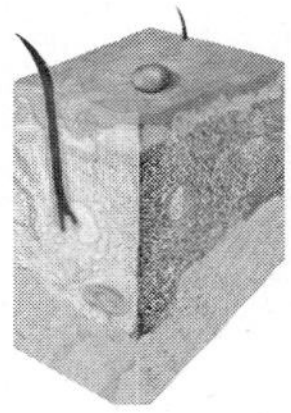	A small elevation on the skin that contains no fluid, but may develop pus
	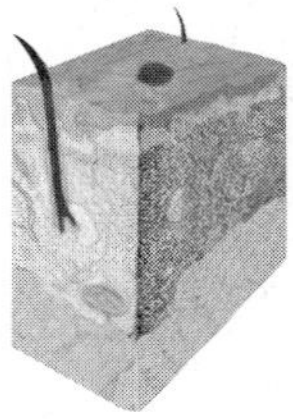	Flat spot or discoloration on the skin

		Small blister or sac containing clear fluid, lying within or just beneath the epidermis
		An itchy, swollen lesion that can be caused by a blow, scratch, bite of an insect, or urticaria (skin allergy), or the sting of a nettle

Secondary Lesions

Fill-in-the-Blank

22 A(n) ______________________ is a thick scar resulting from excessive growth of fibrous tissue.

23 A(n) ______________________ is a skin sore or abrasion produced by scratching or scraping.

24 Severely cracked or chapped lips are an example of a(n) ______________________.

25 Excessive dandruff is an example of a(n) ______________________.

Discuss Disorders of the Sebaceous and Sudoriferous Glands

LO 5 **List and describe disorders of the sebaceous and sudoriferous glands.**

Fill-in-the-Blank/Multiple Choice

26 Identify the disorders in the images below.

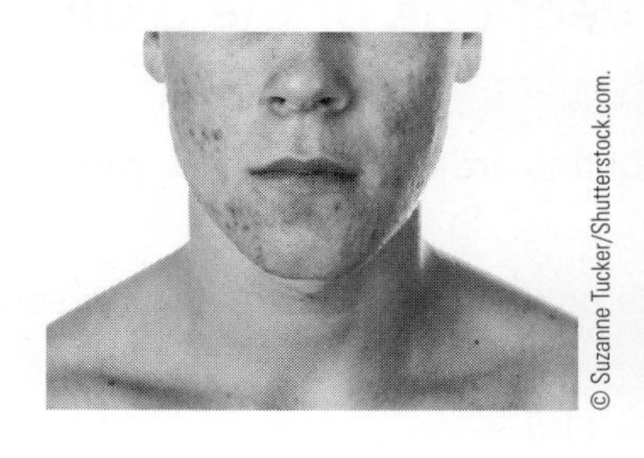

© Suzanne Tucker/Shutterstock.com.

Courtesy Mark Lees Skin Care, Inc.

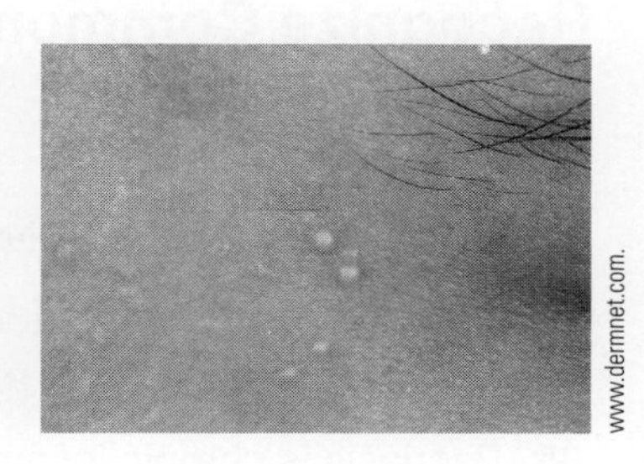

www.dermnet.com.

a. ______________________ **b.** ______________________ **c.** ______________________

27 ______________________ is characterized by flushing, telangiectasis, and, in some cases, the formation of papules and pustules.

a. Rosacea

b. Eczema

c. Milia

d. Acne

28 ______________________ are benign, keratin-filled cysts commonly associated with newborn babies.

a. Rosacea
b. Eczema
c. Milia
d. Acne

29 ______________________ acne is characterized by redness and inflammation with many papules and pustules.

a. Grade I
b. Grade II
c. Grade III
d. Grade IV

30 ______________________ is a deficiency in perspiration that can be life threatening and requires medical attention.

a. Hyperhidrosis
b. Bromhidrosis
c. Anhidrosis
d. Miliaria rubra

31 ______________________ results in foul-smelling perspiration, usually noticeable in the armpits or on the feet.

a. Hyperhidrosis
b. Bromhidrosis
c. Anhidrosis
d. Miliaria rubra

Acne Treatment

Short Answer

32 Briefly describe the basics of acne treatment.

- ____
  ____
- ____
  ____
- ____
  ____

Recognize Common Inflammations and Infections of the Skin

Fill-in-the-Blank

33 ______________________ is not usually chronic if precautions are taken, such as wearing gloves when working with chemicals.

34 Eczema is an inflammatory skin disease that may be acute or chronic in nature and present in many forms of dry or moist ______________________.

35 Psoriasis is chronic inflammatory skin disease characterized by dry red ______________________ covered with coarse, silvery ______________________.

36 Herpes simplex I is a recurring ______________________ infection that produces fever blisters or ______________________ characterized by a single vesicle or group of vesicles with red, swollen bases.

Recognize Pigment Disorders and Hypertrophies of the Skin

LO 6 List and describe types of skin pigmentations.

LO 7 Identify common skin hypertrophies.

Identify Types of Skin Pigmentations

Fill-in-the-Blank

37 Identify the disorders in the images below.

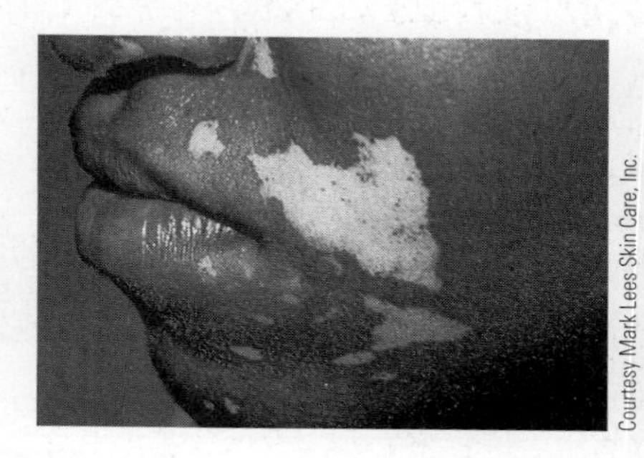

Courtesy Mark Lees Skin Care, Inc.

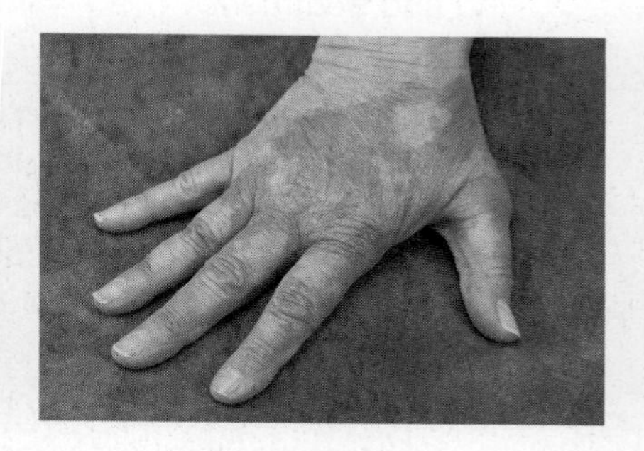

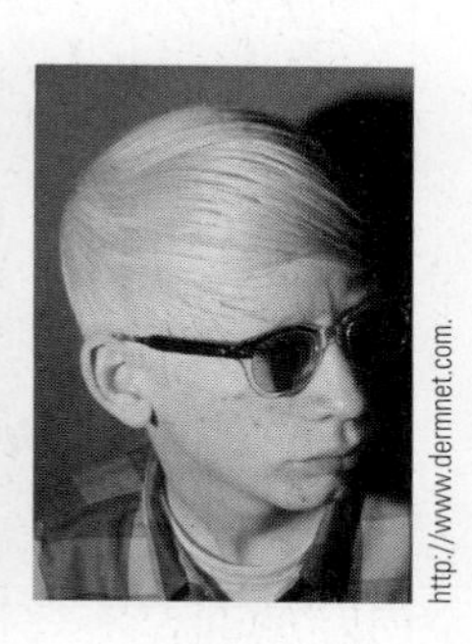

http://www.dermnet.com.

a. ______________ **b.** ______________ **c.** ______________

38 ________________________, also known as the mask of pregnancy, is a condition characterized by hyperpigmentation on the skin in spots that are not elevated.

39 Examples of ________________________ are vitiligo and albinism.

40 A(n) ________________________ is also known as a birthmark.

41 ________________________ is the technical term for freckles, small yellow-colored to brown-colored spots on skin exposed to sunlight and air.

Describe Hypertrophies of the Skin

Matching

42 Match the descriptions with the correct word.

_____ An acquired, superficial, thickened patch of epidermis

_____ Caused by a virus and is infectious

_____ Small brown-colored or flesh-colored outgrowth

_____ Ranges in color from pale tan to brown or bluish black

a. Keratoma

b. Mole

c. Skin tag

d. Verruca (wart)

Understand Skin Cancer

LO 8 **Identify and describe types of skin cancer.**

Fill-in-the-Blank/Case Study

43 Identify the cancer type in the blank column below.

Cancer Type	Description	Image
	Most common and least severe skin cancer; characterized by light or pearly nodules and has a 90% survival rate with early diagnosis and treatment.	
	100% fatal if left untreated—early detection and treatment can result in a 94% 5-year survival rate, which drops drastically, to 62%, once it reaches local lymph nodes; characterized by black or dark brown patches on the skin that may appear uneven in texture, jagged, or raised.	
	Characterized by scaly red papules or nodules. It can spread to other parts of the body; survival rates depend on the stage at diagnosis.	

44 **Assisting Clients with Skin Cancer**

Many people are affected with skin cancer; however, some of them are not aware of it. Barbers are in a unique position to detect some skin cancers and serve clients well when they suspect that their client has skin cancer. Explain how you will use specific information in this chapter to assist you in serving clients suspected of having skin cancer.

____

____

____

____

____

____

____

____

Know How to Maintain the Health of Your Skin

Fill-in-the-Blank

Fill in the terms based on the given definitions.

45 Four factors involved in maintaining the skin's overall health and appearance are ________________, ________________, ________________, and ________________.

46 Some extrinsic factors that influence aging of the skin are ________________, ________________, ________________, and ________________.

Word Review

Fill-in-the-Blank

________________ Congenital leukoderma, or absence of melanin pigment in the body.

________________ A crack in the skin that penetrates to the dermis.

________________ A thick scar resulting from excessive tissue growth.

________________ An open comedone; consists of an accumulation of excess oil (sebum) that has been oxidized to a dark color.

________________ Non-elevated spots due to increased pigmentation in the skin.

________________ A spot or discoloration of the skin, such as a freckle.

________________ The technical name for skin; also another name for the dermis.

________________ An inflammatory skin condition characterized by painful itching; dry or moist lesion forms.

________________ An open skin lesion accompanied by pus and loss of skin depth; a deep erosion; a depression in the skin, normally due to infection or cancer.

________________ Excessive perspiration or sweating.

________________ Chronic congestion of the skin characterized by redness, blood vessel dilation, papules, and pustules.

________________ A skin inflammation caused by exposure to poison ivy, poison oak, or poison sumac.

________________ A structural change in the tissues caused by injury or disease.

________________ The technical name for a birthmark.

________________ Also known as a blackhead; a hair follicle filled with keratin and sebum.

________________ A pimple.

________________ An accumulation of dry or greasy flakes on the skin.

________________ An abnormal cell mass resulting from excessive multiplication of cells.

CHAPTER 10

PROPERTIES AND DISORDERS OF THE HAIR AND SCALP

LEARNING OBJECTIVES

After completing this chapter, you will be able to:

LO1 Identify and distinguish the different structures of the hair root.

LO2 Identify and distinguish the three layers of the hair shaft.

LO3 Identify and explain the three types of side bonds of the cortex.

LO4 Name and describe the three phases of the hair growth cycle.

LO5 Identify and define seven types of hair loss.

LO6 Identify and describe two FDA approved treatments for hair loss.

LO7 Identify and define common hair disorders.

LO8 Define common scalp disorders and identify those requiring medical attention.

LO9 Identify the factors to be observed and considered during a hair and scalp analysis.

Introduction

Short Answer/Fill-in-the-Blank

1 List the reasons why studying properties and disorders of the hair and scalp is important for a barber.

a. ______________________________

____

b. ______________________________

____

c. ______________________________

____

2 The scientific study of hair, its disorders, and its care is called ______________________.

3 List the functions of the hair.

a. ______________________________

____

b. ______________________________

____

c. ______________________________

____

Why Study Properties and Disorders of the Hair and Scalp?

Multiple Choice

4 Barbers should have a thorough understanding of properties and disorders of the hair and scalp because:

a. They need to know the difference between what is normal and abnormal.

b. It will be easier to make hair grow fast.

c. They need to test new products on clients.

d. Scientists will interview them to find cures.

Discover the Structure of Hair

LO 1 **Identify and distinguish the different structures of the hair root.**

LO 2 **Identify and distinguish the three layers of the hair shaft.**

Structures of the Hair Root

Fill-in-the-Blank/Labeling

5 Sometimes, more than one hair will grow from a single ____________________.

6 The lower part of the hair ____________________ is hollow and fits over and covers the dermal papilla.

7 Strong emotions or cold causes the ____________________ to contract, which makes the hair stand up straight, resulting in goose bumps.

8 The ____________________ contains the blood and nerve supply that provides the nutrients needed for hair growth.

9 Label the structures of the hair.

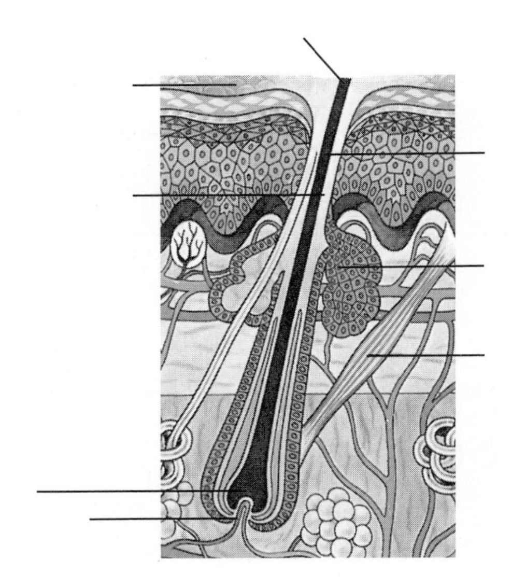

Structures of the Hair Shaft

Multiple Choice

10 The medulla layer of the hair may be absent in ______________________ hair.

a. very fine　　**c.** straight

b. extremely curly　　**d.** red

11 The ______________________ layer provides a barrier that protects the inner structure of the hair.

a. medulla　　**c.** cuticle

b. cortex　　**d.** papilla

12 The cortex is the ______________________ layer of the hair.

a. innermost　　**c.** middle

b. outermost　　**d.** spiny

Learn about the Chemical Composition of Hair

LO 3 **Identify and explain the three types of side bonds of the cortex.**

Fill-in-the-Blank

13 Hair is composed of the protein ______________________.

14 Protein is made of chemical units called ______________________.

15 The spiral shape of a coiled protein is called a ______________________.

Side Bonds of the Hair Cortex

Fill-in-the-Blank

16 Identify the bond of the hair in the blank column based on the descriptions below.

Bond	Strength	Broken By	Re-formed By
	Weak; physical	Changes in pH	Normalizing pH
	Strong; chemical	Thio perms and thio relaxers	Oxidation with neutralizer
	Weak; physical	Water or heat	Drying or cooling

17 Although individual hydrogen bonds are weak, they are so numerous in the hair that they account for about ______________ of the hair's overall strength.

18 ______________ heat can break disulfide bonds.

Hair Pigment and Wave Pattern

Fill-in-the-Blank

19 Natural hair color is the result of the melanin pigment found within the ______________.

20 There are two types of melanin: ______________ and ______________. All natural color is dependent on the ______________ of one to the other.

21 The ______________ of hair refers to the shape of the hair strand and is described as ______________, ______________, ______________, and ______________.

Discuss Hair Growth

LO 4 **Name and describe the three phases of the hair growth cycle.**

Matching

22 Match the correct type of hair with each description.

_____ Almost never has a medulla or melanin		**a. Terminal hair**
_____ Long, coarse hair		**b. Vellus hair**
_____ Also called lanugo		
_____ Helps in evaporation of perspiration		
_____ Usually found on the scalp, legs, arms, and body		

Growth Cycles of Hair and Hair Shedding

Multiple Choice

23 About ______________ percent of scalp hair exists in the anagen phase.

a. 60 | **c.** 80
b. 70 | **d.** 90

24 What does *not* occur during the catagen phase?

a. The follicle shrinks.
b. The hair bulb disappears.
c. The hair sheds.
d. The root end forms a rounded club.

25 The telogen phase lasts for approximately ______________ or until the hair is shed.

a. 24 hours
b. 1 to 2 weeks
c. 3 to 6 months
d. 4 to 5 years

26 The only treatments that have been scientifically proven to increase hair growth are minoxidil and ______________.

a. singeing
b. finasteride
c. massage
d. essential oils

27 It is normal to lose an average of ______________ hairs per day.

a. 15 to 30
b. 50 to 60
c. 75 to 100
d. 100 to 150

Growth Patterns

Short Answer

28 Briefly describe these common growth patterns.

a. Whorl: ______________

____

____

____

b. Hair Stream: ______________

____

____

____

c. Cowlick: ______________

____

____

____

Understand Hair Loss

LO 5 Identify and define seven types of hair loss.

LO 6 Identify and describe two FDA approved treatments for hair loss.

Identify Types of Abnormal Hair Loss

Matching/Fill-in-the-Blank

29 Match the description with the type of hair loss.

_____ Total scalp hair loss	**a. Androgenic alopecia**
_____ Occurring in old age and is permanent	**b. Alopecia premature**
_____ May occur on the scalp and elsewhere on the body	**c. Alopecia areata**
_____ An autoimmune disorder	**d. Alopecia totalis**
_____ Known as male pattern baldness	**e. Alopecia universalis**
_____ Non-inflamed bald areas look molted	**f. Alopecia senilis**
_____ Can begin as early as in the teens	**g. Alopecia syphilitica**

30 Almost ____________________ percent of men and women show some degree of hair loss by age ____________________.

31 With ____________________, the hair usually grows back once the disease is cured.

Describe Hair Loss Treatments

Multiple Choice/Case Study

32 Which of the following is a possible side effect of finasteride?

a. Depression.
b. Overactive bladder.
c. Weight loss.
d. Weight gain.

33 With proper training, barbers can ____________________ to camouflage hair loss.

a. offer hair weaves
b. prescribe Propecia®
c. perform a hair transplant
d. prescribe finasteride

34 Barber's Choice of Hair Loss Treatment

Most clients trust their barber and come seeking advice, including for hair loss treatment. Of the available treatments for hair loss (i.e., Rogaine, Theroxidil, Minoxidil, Propecia, or hair transplant), which would you recommend for a 35-year-old man who suffers mild hair loss? What would your recommendation be based on? What would be the next step to take toward treatment?

____

____

____

____

Recognize Disorders of the Hair and Scalp

LO 7 Identify and define common hair disorders.

LO 8 Define common scalp disorders and identify those requiring medical attention.

Recognize Disorders of the Hair

Matching

35 Review the following hair disorders, then match each with the correct technical term from the list.

_____ Gray hair	**a. Hypertrichosis**
_____ Exists at or before birth	**b. Trichoptilosis**
_____ Alternating bands of gray and pigmented hair	**c. Trichorrhexis nodosa**
_____ Abnormal growth of terminal hair	**d. Canities**
_____ Develops with age and the result of genetics	**e. Monilethrix**
_____ Knotted hair	**f. Acquired canities**
_____ Split ends	**g. Congenital canities**
_____ Beaded hair	**h. Fragilitas crinium**
_____ Brittle hair	**i. Ringed hair**

Identify Disorders of the Scalp: Dandruff

Fill-in-the-Blank

36 _______________ is the technical term for dandruff. Current research confirms that dandruff is the result of a fungus called _______________.

37 Anti-dandruff shampoos can be recommended to a client with _______________ conditions, but _______________ cases should be referred to a physician.

38 Identify the disorder in the blank space provided.

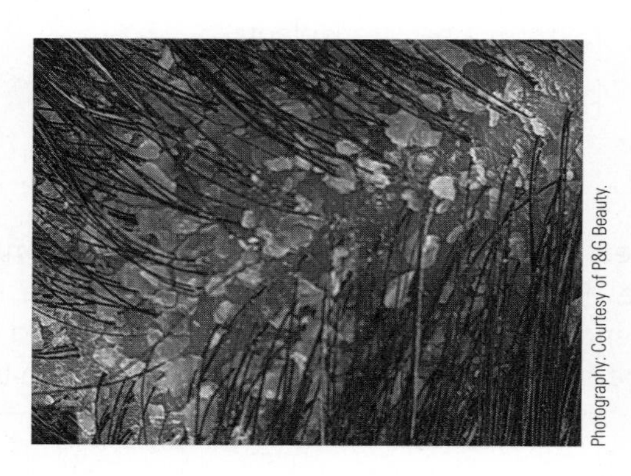

Photography: Courtesy of P&G Beauty.

a. _______________

Photography: Courtesy of P&G Beauty.

b. _______________

Identify Fungal Infections: Tinea

Fill-in-the-Blank

39 ________________________ is caused by fungal organisms and is characterized by itching, scales, and, sometimes, painful circular lesions.

40 Infected skin scales or hair containing the fungi are known to spread tinea; ________________________, ________________________, and unclean personal articles (such as brushes) are also sources of transmission.

41 ________________________ begins as small, round, slightly scaly, inflamed patches that enlarge, clearing up somewhat at the center with elevation at the borders.

42 ________________________ is characterized by dry, sulfur-yellow, cuplike crusts on the scalp having a peculiar, musty odor.

Recognize Parasitic Infestations and Bacterial Infections

Multiple Choice

43 Pediculosis capitis is the infestation of the hair and scalp with ________________________.

a. ringworm	**c.** scabies
b. head lice	**d.** fungus

44 ________________________, or barber's itch, is an infection of the hair follicles characterized by inflamed pustules in the bearded areas of the face and neck.

a. Scabies	**c.** Folliculitis barbae
b. Sycosis barbae	**d.** Pseudofolliculitis barbae

45 A ________________________ is an acute bacterial infection of a hair follicle, producing constant pain.

a. furuncle	**c.** malassezia
b. tinea	**d.** sycosis

Learn How to Perform a Hair and Scalp Analysis

LO 9 **Identify the factors to be observed and considered during a hair and scalp analysis.**

Short Answer

46 Describe how and what knowledge can be gained through using the following senses:

a. Sight: ____

____

____

____

b. Hearing: ____________________

____

____

____

c. Smell: ____________________

____

____

____

d. Touch: ____________________

____

____

____

47 What disorders or conditions might you find in the scalp analysis that would prompt you to suspend the service or exercise caution?

____

____

____

____

____

Perform a Hair Analysis

Matching

48 Match the correct texture of hair with each description.

_____ Standard texture	**a. Coarse**
_____ Largest diameter	**b. Medium**
_____ Hard, glassy finish	**c. Fine**
_____ Smallest diameter	**d. Wiry**
_____ Easier to process	
_____ Cuticle scales lie flat against hair shaft	
_____ More difficult for products to penetrate	
_____ Most common	

Hair Density and Porosity

Short Answer/Fill-in-the-Blank

49 Describe how hair density is classified and what it depends upon.

____

____

____

50 Describe how to check the porosity of hair.

____

____

____

51 Describe how resistant (low porosity) hair feels.

____

____

____

52 Determine whether each hair strand in the images below has low, average, or high porosity.

The Gillette Research Institute.

The Gillette Research Institute.

The Gillette Research Institute.

a. ____________ **b.** ____________ **c.** ____________

Hair Elasticity

Fill-in-the-Blank

53 Hair that breaks easily or fails to return to its normal length has ____________ elasticity.

54 ____________ hair may stretch up to 50 percent of its original length and return to that length without breaking.

Word Review

Matching

Draw a line connecting each term with its description.

Alopecia senilis	The result of an acute, deep-seated bacterial infection in the subcutaneous tissue.
Carbuncle	Small, cone-shaped elevation located at the base of the hair follicle that fits into the hair bulb.
Dermal papilla	Hair loss occurring in old age.
Eumelanin	Hair that grows in a circular pattern.
Follicle	A tube-like depression in the skin that contains the hair root.
Hair bulb	Soft, downy hair that appears on the body.
Keratin	Also known as cross bonds; hydrogen, salt, and sulfur bonds in the hair cortex.
Lanugo	The protein of which hair is formed.
Medulla	End bonds; chemical bonds that join amino acids end to end.
Peptide bonds	Vellus hair.
Side bonds	The innermost or center layer of the hair shaft.
Tinea	A club-shaped structure that forms the lower part of the hair root.
Vellus hair	The technical name for ringworm.
Whorl	Melanin that gives brown and black color to hair.

CHAPTER 11

TREATMENT OF THE HAIR AND SCALP

LEARNING OBJECTIVES

After completing this chapter, you will be able to:

LO1 Discuss the benefits of a shampoo service.

LO2 Select products for different hair types and textures.

LO3 Describe proper draping procedures for various services.

LO4 Identify basic considerations for performing a shampoo service.

LO5 Describe two shampooing methods.

LO6 Discuss reasons why a client may find fault with a shampoo service.

LO7 Describe scalp massage manipulations and techniques.

LO8 Explain services that may be included in a hair or scalp treatment.

Introduction

Fill-in-the-Blank

1 The treatment of the hair and scalp includes ______________________, ______________________, ______________________, and special treatments for hair and scalp conditions.

2 When performed correctly, barbering services are ______________________.

Why Study Treatment of the Hair and Scalp?

Short Answer

3 List the reasons why studying treatment of the hair and scalp is important for a barber.

a. ____

____

____

b. ____

____

____

c. ____

____

____

Discuss the Shampoo Service

LO 1 **Discuss the benefits of a shampoo service.**

LO 2 **Select products for different hair types and textures.**

Review Shampoos and Conditioners

Fill-in-the-Blank

4 The purpose of a shampoo product and service is to ______________________ the scalp and hair.

5 Since shampoos do not contain the harsh ______________________ found in soaps and detergents, they leave the hair in a more manageable condition.

6 Hair conditioners typically range from ______________________ on the pH scale.

7 Shampoos are ______________________ emulsions with a pH range of ______________________.

8 Fill in the table below with one product that best matches each combination of hair type and texture.

Hair Type	**Hair Texture**		
	Fine	**Medium**	**Coarse**
Straight			
Wavy, curly, extremely curly			
Dry and damaged			

Know How to Drape

LO 3 **Describe proper draping procedures for various services.**

Fill-in-the-Blank

9 ______________________ capes are waterproof drapes made of vinyl that are used to protect the client's skin and clothing from water, liquids, and chemical processes.

10 ______________________ capes are made of nylon or other synthetic materials.

Learn Draping Methods

Short Answer

11 Describe the draping procedures for the following services.

a. Chemical service:

____

____

____

____

____

b. Shampoo service:

____

____

____

____

____

c. Mustache/beard trim service:

____

____

____

____

____

d. Haircut service:

____

____

____

____

____

Understand the Shampoo Service

LO 4 **Identify basic considerations for performing a shampoo service.**

LO 5 **Describe two shampooing methods.**

LO 6 **Discuss reasons why a client may find fault with a shampoo service.**

Short Answer/Fill-in-the-Blank

12 List the basic considerations for performing a shampoo service.

a. ____

____

b. ____

____

c. ____

____

13 Typically, the barber stands ____________________ the client and shampoo bowl when performing the shampoo.

Describe Two Methods of Shampooing and Rinsing

Fill-in-the-Blank

14 The ____________________ method of shampooing is favored because it is more comfortable for the client and permits greater speed and efficiency by the barber.

15 Write the correct shampoo method in the blank for the images below.

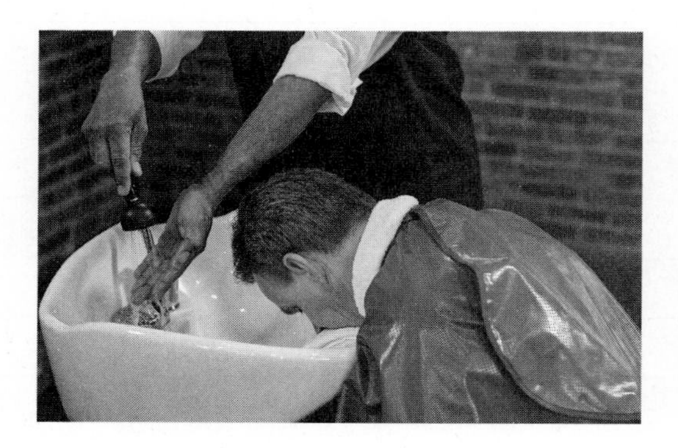

a. ____________________

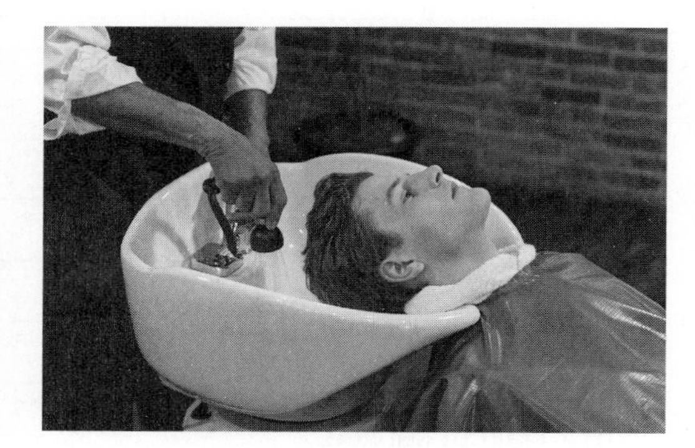

b. ____________________

Shampooing Clients with Special Needs

Short Answer/Fill-in-the-Blank/Matching

16 Good posture at the shampoo sink helps to prevent muscle aches, back strain, and fatigue. List four suggestions to help maintain a good posture while shampooing.

a. ____

____

b. ____

____

c. ____

____

d. ____

____

17 Complete the list of reasons a client may find fault with a shampoo service.

- Improper ____________________ selection
- ____________________ scalp massage
- ____________________ water temperatures
- Shampoo or water that runs onto client's ____________________, ____________________, or ____________________
- ____________________ or soiling the client's clothing
- ____________________ or ____________________ the client's scalp
- Improper hair ____________________
- Insufficient cleansing and ____________________

18 Match the correct characteristic of the scalp and hair with its possible findings when analyzed.

_____ Dry, oily, normal, and/or presence of abrasions or disorders

_____ Dry, brittle, fragile, oily, normal, or chemically treated

_____ Thin, medium, thick

_____ Fine, average, coarse

_____ Low (resistant), average (normal), high (overly porous)

_____ Low (breaks easily), average (normal)

a. Hair density

b. Hair porosity

c. Hair texture

d. Hair condition

e. Scalp condition

f. Hair elasticity

19 Fill in the blanks to complete the steps used in the shampoo service.

1. ____________________ the client for the shampoo service.

2. ____________________ with the client about products, hair and scalp problems, or any questions the client has about his hair or scalp.

3. ______________________ the condition of the client's hair and scalp. Use ______________________ movement to lightly ______________________ the scalp to loosen epidermal scales, debris, and scalp tissues.

4. ______________________ the client for the shampoo service. ______________________ the client while draping the back of the cape over the back of the chair.

5. Saturate the hair with ______________________ water, protecting the ______________________ and ______________________ against splashes. ______________________ the head while saturating the nape and back sections.

6. Apply ______________________ to all parts of the scalp.

7. Starting at the ______________________ hairline, work along the sides toward the back and nape areas to massage and produce a ______________________. Use ______________________ movements over the entire head area to massage the scalp for several minutes. Repeat these movements over the top, side, and back sections several times.

8. Remove excess lather with a ______________________ of the palm from the front of the head to the back; ______________________ hair thoroughly with warm water using a moderate to strong spray.

9. Apply ______________________, massage through hair, and rinse thoroughly.

10. ______________________ the hair.

11. Raise the client to a ______________________ position and lightly ______________________ the hair; wipe the face and ears if necessary.

12. ______________________ the hair into position for cutting.

Learn about Scalp and Hair Treatments

LO 7 **Describe scalp massage manipulations and techniques.**

LO 8 **Explain services that may be included in a hair or scalp treatment.**

Explain Scalp Massage Manipulations

Multiple Choice

20 Which of the following is *not* an effect of a proper massage manipulation?

- **a.** Increased blood flow.
- **b.** Soothed nerves.
- **c.** Lower blood pressure.
- **d.** More flexible scalp.

21 A scalp massage as part of a scalp treatment most often includes ______________________ massage movements.

- **a.** rotary and sliding
- **b.** scratching
- **c.** highly pressured
- **d.** squeezing

22 Massage manipulations should be ______________________.

- **a.** fast and short
- **b.** slow and long
- **c.** fast and rhythmic
- **d.** slow and rhythmic

23 Which of the following does *not* help to stimulate muscles, nerves, and blood vessels in the scalp area?

- **a.** Length of the fingers.
- **b.** Balls of the fingertips.
- **c.** Cushions of the palms.
- **d.** Tips of the fingernails.

Describe Scalp and Hair Treatments

Case Study/Short Answer

24 Explaining a Scalp Treatment

Clients often see a barber when they are having problems with their hair or scalp that they themselves cannot fix. However, they may be reluctant to have a service performed, especially if they do not know what is involved. Imagine that a client tells you that he is having problems with dry scalp and dandruff and wants treatment. Explain the service(s) you would perform to help relieve the client's condition.

____

____

____

____

____

____

____

____

____

____

25 What can be used for a scalp steam if a scalp steamer is unavailable?

____

____

____

____

____

____

____

____

____

____

26 Fill in the steps for a hair tonic treatment below.

1. ______________________________
2. ______________________________
3. ______________________________
4. ______________________________
5. ______________________________

Word Review

Word Scramble

Unscramble each key term, using the provided definitions as clues.

pnigard ______________________________

The term used to describe the covering of the client's clothing with a cape for sanitation and protection.

raih renoitidnoc ______________________________

A product designed to moisturize the hair or restore some of the hair's oils or proteins.

apcls noitieridcno ______________________________

A cream or ointment-based product used to soften or treat the scalp.

acpls atems ______________________________

The process of using steam towels or a steaming unit to soften and open scalp pores.

maoposh ______________________________

A hair and scalp cleansing product.

CHAPTER 12

MEN'S FACIAL MASSAGE AND TREATMENTS

LEARNING OBJECTIVES

After completing this chapter, you will be able to:

LO1 **List the modalities that affect muscle action.**

LO2 **Know the muscles of the scalp, face, and neck.**

LO3 **List the modalities that affect nerve responses.**

LO4 **Know the main cranial nerve branches of the scalp, face, and neck.**

LO5 **Identify arteries and veins affected by facial massage.**

LO6 **Describe the physiological effects of massage.**

LO7 **Name and describe massage manipulations.**

LO8 **Explain the use of facial and electrotherapy equipment.**

LO9 **Identify skin types, facial treatments, and products.**

Introduction

Short Answer/Fill-in-the-Blank

1 List the reasons why studying men's facial massage and treatments is important for a barber.

a. ______________________________

____

b. ______________________________

____

c. ______________________________

____

2 Male clients represent about ______________ percent of the skin clientele in spas and salons.

3 Historically, ______________ and ______________ facials were standard customer services performed by the barber.

Why Study Men's Facial Massage and Treatments?

Multiple Choice

4 Barbers should have a thorough understanding of men's facial massage and treatments because:

a. Salons and spas are all going out of business.

b. Clients want to know how to do facial massages at home.

c. Men are no longer interested in having their hair cut.

d. Barbers need to be competent in all of the services for which they are licensed to perform.

Review Subdermal Systems

LO 1 **List the modalities that affect muscle action.**

LO 2 **Know the muscles of the scalp, face, and neck.**

LO 3 **List the modalities that affect nerve responses.**

LO 4 **Know the main cranial nerve branches of the scalp, face, and neck.**

LO 5 **Identify arteries and veins affected by facial massage.**

Matching

5 Match the correct subdermal system with the descriptions below.

_____	Long, white, fibrous cords that act as message carriers from the brain and spinal column to and from all parts of the body		**a. Muscles**
_____	Thin-walled vessels that contain valves that keep the blood flowing to the heart and prevent it from flowing backward		**b. Nerves**
_____	Elastic, thick-walled blood vessels that transport blood under high pressure		**c. Arteries**
_____	Fibrous tissues that have the ability to stretch and contract to product all body movements		**d. Veins**
_____	Not directly associated with the performance of facial treatments		

Describe the Modalities That Affect Muscle Action

Short Answer

6 List the modalities associated with facials.

- ______________________________
- ______________________________
- ______________________________
- ______________________________

- ______________________________
- ______________________________
- ______________________________

Discuss the Muscles Affected by Facial Massage

Fill-in-the-Blank

7 When performing a facial massage, you will be concerned with the voluntary muscles of the ______________________, and ______________________.

8 Write the muscle that matches the description. Complete the table of muscles below.

Muscle	Location	Description and Function
	Neck	Muscle that extends from the collar and chest bones to the temporal bone in back of the ear that bends and rotates the head
	Scalp	Muscle at the front portion of the epicranius that draws scalp forward and causes wrinkles across the forehead
	Scalp	Tendon that connects the occipitalis and frontalis
	Eyebrows	Muscle that surrounds the eye socket and closes the eyelid
	Mouth	Muscle on both sides of the face that extends from the zygomatic bone to the upper lip and that pulls the mouth upward, inward, and backward, for example, when smiling
	Nose	Muscle that covers the top of the nose, depresses the eyebrow, and causes wrinkles across the bridge of nose; other nasal muscles contract and expand the openings of the nostrils
	Scalp	Muscle at the back part of the epicranius that draws the scalp backward
	Mouth	Thin, flat muscle between the upper and lower jaws; compresses the cheeks and expels air between the lips
	Mouth	Muscle surrounding the upper lip that elevates the upper lip and dilates the nostrils, for example, when expressing distaste
	Ears	Muscle behind the ear that draws the ear backward
	Mouth	Muscle on both sides of the face that extends from the zygomatic bone to the angle of the mouth that pulls the mouth upward and backward, for example, when laughing or smiling
	Mouth	Muscle that raises angle of mouth and draws it inward
	Mouth	Muscle at the tip of the chin that elevates the lower lip and raises and wrinkles the skin of the chin

	Mouth	Muscle that surrounds the lower part of the lip, depresses the lower lip, and draws it to one side, for example, when expressing sarcasm
	Mouth	Muscle that extends from the masseter muscle to the angle of the mouth that draws the corner of the mouth out and back, for example, when grinning
	Mouth	Flat band of muscle around the upper and lower lips that compresses, contracts, puckers, and wrinkles the lips
	Neck	Broad muscle extending from the chest and shoulder muscles to the side of the chin; responsible for depressing the lower jaw and lip
	Mouth	Muscle that extends along the side of the chin that draws the corner of the mouth down
	Mastication muscles	Muscles that coordinate opening and closing mouth; chewing muscles
	Ears	Muscle above the ear that draws the ear upward
	Neck	Muscle that covers the back of the neck allowing movement of the shoulders
	Ears	Muscle in front of the ear that draws the ear forward
	Scalp	Broad muscle that covers the top of the skull
	Eyebrows	Muscle beneath the frontalis and orbicularis oculi that draws the eyebrows down and in and wrinkles the forehead vertically

Discuss the Modalities That Affect Nerve Responses

Fill-in-the-Blank/Short Answer

9 ______________ stimulation causes muscles to ______________ and ______________.

10 Heat and ______________ on the skin cause ______________ and cold causes ______________.

11 List the means by which nerves may be stimulated.

- ______________
- ______________
- ______________
- ______________
- ______________
- ______________

Discuss the Main Cranial Nerves Affected by Facial Massage

Multiple Choice

12 How many pairs of cranial nerves exist?

a. 12.
b. 8.
c. 30.
d. 6.

13 Which cranial nerve is the chief sensory nerve of the face?

a. Fifth cranial nerve.
b. Seventh cranial nerve.
c. Ninth cranial nerve.
d. Eleventh cranial nerve.

14 Which cranial nerve is the motor nerve that controls motions of the neck muscles?

a. Fifth cranial nerve.
b. Seventh cranial nerve.
c. Ninth cranial nerve.
d. Eleventh cranial nerve.

15 The ____________________ nerves originate at the spinal cord and their branches supply the muscles and scalp at the back of the head and neck.

a. accessory
b. cervical
c. facial
d. trigeminal

Discuss Arteries and Veins Affected by Facial Massage

Fill-in-the-Blank/Matching

16 Arteries are vessels that transport ____________________ from the heart to all parts of the body.

17 The ____________________ from the head, face, and neck returns to the heart through the internal jugular and external jugular ____________________ of the neck.

18 Match the correct primary artery with each definition.

_____ A continuation of external carotid, supplies muscles, skin, and scalp on the front, side, and top of the head.

_____ The main sources of blood supply to the head, face, and neck; located at the sides of the neck.

_____ Supplies the scalp and back of the head up to the crown.

_____ Supplies the scalp behind and above the ear.

_____ Supplies the lower region of the face, mouth, and nose.

a. Common carotids
b. External maxillary
c. Superficial temporal
d. Occipital
e. Posterior auricular

Understand the Theory of Massage

LO 6 **Describe the physiological effects of massage.**

LO 7 **Name and describe massage manipulations.**

Fill-in-the-Blank

19 Facial massage involves the ______________ or ______________ external manipulation of the ______________ and ______________.

20 Benefits to be gained from massage will depend on the type of massage ______________ used; amount of ______________ used; ______________ of the movement; and ______________ of the massage manipulation.

Discuss the Physiological Effects of Massage

Short Answer

21 How does the part being massaged react?

____

____

22 List four benefits obtained by receiving a massage.

- ____
  ____
- ____
  ____
- ____
  ____
- ____
  ____

Know about Massage Manipulations

Fill-in-the-Blank

23 A ______________ is a point on the skin where nerves that control the underlying ______________ are located.

24 When ______________ stimulation is applied to a nerve, the muscle responds by ______________.

25 A ______________ is a tender area in a muscle caused by a localized ______________ or ______________ in the muscle fiber that can radiate pain to other locations in the body.

26 When used in a facial massage, ______________ but ______________ pressure can be applied to a trigger point for about ______________, followed by stroking movements to help relieve painful areas.

Massage Manipulations

Matching

27 Match the correct massage movement to the description.

_____	Pressure is applied on the skin with the fingers or palms while moving over an underlying structure		**a. Friction**
_____	Stroking movement		**b. Percussion**
_____	Performed with light, firm pressure		**c. Effleurage**
_____	Rapid shaking movement		**d. Vibration**
_____	Exerts an invigorating effect on the area being massaged		**e. Pétrissage**
_____	Most stimulating form of massage		
_____	Short, quick tapping, slapping, or hacking movements		
_____	Light, continuous movement that should be applied in a slow and rhythmic manner over the skin, with no pressure		
_____	Deep rubbing movement		
_____	Should be used sparingly and not exceed a few seconds' duration on any one area		
_____	Frequently used to apply lotions or creams		
_____	Uses the fingertips or an electric massager or vibrator		
_____	Kneading movement		
_____	Proven to be beneficial to the circulation and glandular activity of the skin		

Guidelines for Performing Facial Massage Manipulations

Fill-in-the-Blank/Short Answer

28 When massaging areas of the head, face, or neck, any pressure employed should be applied in a(n) ______________________ direction.

29 Perform massage manipulations ______________________ and ______________________.

30 The ______________________ of a muscle is the attachment point to a movable bone and the ______________________ of a muscle is the attachment point to an immovable bone.

31 How does the presence of facial hair change the approach to facial manipulations on the face?

____

____

32 List the conditions which contraindicate recommending or performing massage.

- ______________________________
- ______________________________
- ______________________________
- ______________________________
- ______________________________

Know the Purpose of Facial Equipment

LO 8 **Explain the use of facial and electrotherapy equipment.**

Identify Facial Appliances

Matching

33 Match the correct facial appliance with each description.

_____ An electrical appliance with interchangeable brushes that attach to the rotating head of the unit

_____ Do not use over the upper lip, as it may cause discomfort

_____ An electrical appliance that produces and projects moist, uniform steam that can be positioned over sections of the head or face for softening and cleansing purpose

_____ Should never be used on skin that has been treated with Retin-A®

_____ A handheld unit that transmits vibrations through the barber's hand and fingertips to the client's skin and muscles

_____ Ensures a ready supply of warm towels for facial services

_____ Softens the skin, increases perspiration, and softens accumulations in the follicles

a. Electric massager

b. Brush machine

c. Hot-towel cabinet

d. Facial steamer

Identify Electrotherapy Equipment

Fill-in-the-Blank

34 Facial treatments performed with facial machines that produce electrical ______________________ are a form of ______________________.

35 The two modalities most often used in facial treatments are ______________________ and ______________________.

Electrodes

Fill-in-the-Blank

36 Each modality requires an electrode to ________________ and ________ the current to the client's skin.

37 The ____________________ appliance requires only one electrode. ________ machines have two electrodes.

38 A(n) ____________________ is red with a plus sign (+) and a(n) ____________________ is black with a minus sign (–).

High-Frequency Machine

Fill-in-the-Blank/Short Answer

39 High-frequency current is also known as ____________________, and sometimes called the ____________________ because of its color.

40 The primary actions of high-frequency current are ____________________ and ____________________.

41 When performing electrotherapy treatments, the barber and the client must avoid contact with ____________________ or ____________________.

42 The electrodes for high-frequency machines are made of ____________________ or ____________________.

43 For general facial or scalp treatments, no more than ____________________ of high-frequency treatment should be allowed.

44 List the many benefits of using a high-frequency machine.

- ____________________
- ____________________
- ____________________
- ____________________
- ____________________
- ____________________

45 List three client conditions that contraindicate using high-frequency current.

- ____________________
  ____
- ____________________
  ____
- ____________________
  ____

High-Frequency Application Methods

Fill-in-the-Blank

46 The two primary methods for applying high-frequency current are ______________________ and ______________________.

47 Direct surface application is performed for its ______________________ and ______________________ effect on the skin.

48 Direct surface application can be used on ______________________ skin, over facial ______________________, or over ______________________ for a sparking effect.

49 The high-frequency machine produces a ______________________ effect that stimulates ______________________ and has an ______________________ effect on the skin.

50 Indirect application is performed with the client ______________________ the wire glass electrode ______________________.

51 To prevent shock, the power is turned on ________________ the client holds the electrode firmly and turned off ________________ the electrode is removed from the client's hand.

52 Indirect application of the current produces both a ___________ and ___________ effect on the skin and is ideal for ______________________ or ______________________ skin.

53 When using high-frequency current, never use a skin or scalp lotion that contains ______________________ prior to the electrical treatment.

Galvanic Machine

Fill-in-the-Blank

54 Galvanic current can be used to produce chemical ______________________ and ionic ______________________ reactions in the skin.

55 Galvanic current is beneficial for _________ skin and _________.

56 The most popular electrodes for the galvanic machine are the ______________________ and the ______________________.

Galvanic Current Reactions

Matching

57 Match the correct term with each description.

_____	Penetrates an alkaline-PH product into the skin	**a. Desincrustation**
_____	Causes a chemical reaction that helps emulsify or liquefy sebum for easy extraction	**b. Iontophoresis**
_____	The same electrode can also be used to close follicles, decrease redness, prevent inflammation, soothe nerves, and harden tissues	**c. Cataphoresis**
_____	Requires an acid-based solution applied to the skin	**d. Anaphoresis**
_____	Uses galvanic current to force water-soluble solutions into the skin	
_____	Introduces an acid-PH product into the skin	
_____	Facilitates deep pore cleansing	
_____	The same electrode can also be used to stimulate circulation to dry skin, stimulate nerves, and soften tissues	

Microcurrent

Fill-in-the-Blank

58 Microcurrent is a type of ______________ that uses a very low level of electrical current.

59 Microcurrent is best known for ______________ the skin and producing a ______________ on aging skin, which lacks elasticity.

Microdermabrasion

Multiple Choice

60 Microdermabrasion is a method of ______________ the skin's surface.

a. tightening
b. exfoliating
c. hydrating
d. bleaching

61 Microdermabrasion can be used to treat ______________.

a. acne
b. oily skin
c. dry skin
d. wrinkles

Light Therapy

Fill-in-the-Blank/Short Answer

62 Light therapy is the process of using ______________ to treat certain conditions of the ______________ and ______________.

63 ______________, ______________, and ______________ are used to produce different therapeutic effects on the skin.

64 What effects are created by the type of ultraviolet bulb used?

- UVA rays – ______________
- UVB rays – ______________
- UVC rays – ______________

65 Ultraviolet lamps may be used to treat ______________, or ______________ conditions.

66 List the effects that ultraviolet lamps may produce.

- ______________
- ______________
- ______________
- ______________

67 An ultraviolet lamp should be positioned ______________ from the skin.

68 Average exposure to UV rays may produce ______________; overdoses can cause ______________.

69 Infrared rays generally produce a soothing and beneficial type of heat that extends for some distance into the tissues of the body. List the effects of the infrared rays on the skin.

- ______________________
- ______________________
- ______________________
- ______________________
- ______________________

70 Do not allow infrared rays to remain on a skin area for more than ______________.

71 Total exposure time to infrared rays should not exceed ______________.

Contraindications for Electrotherapy

Short Answer

72 List the contraindicating conditions for electrotherapy.

- ______________________
- ______________________
- ______________________
- ______________________
- ______________________
- ______________________
- ______________________
- ______________________
- ______________________
- ______________________
- ______________________

Review Safety Precautions for Using Electrical Equipment

Fill-in-the-Blank

73 ______________ any appliances when they are not being used.

74 Avoid getting cords ______________.

75 ______________ and ______________ all electrodes properly.

76 ______________ the client at all times.

77 Do not allow the client to touch ______________ while electrical treatments are being performed.

78 Do not leave the ______________ while the client is attached to an ______________.

79 Do not touch two metallic objects at the same time while connected to an ______________.

80 Carelessness can result in ______________ or ______________.

Learn about Facial Treatments

LO 9 **Identify skin types, facial treatments, and products.**

Fill-in-the-Blank

81 Facials in the barbershop are considered to be either ______________ or ______________ treatments.

82 ______________ help maintain the health of facial skin through correct cleansing, toning, and massage.

83 ______________ correct skin conditions such as dryness, oiliness, blackheads, aging lines, and minor acne.

Describe Skin Types

Short Answer/Matching

84 What is skin type based on?

____

____

____

85 Match the correct skin type to each description.

____ Characterized by excess sebum production and may appear shiny or greasy

____ Maintenance and preservative care is the goal of treatment

____ Water-based products work best

____ Does not produce enough sebum to prevent the evaporation of cell moisture

____ Requires more cleansing and exfoliation than other types

____ Can be both oily and dry in different areas of the face

____ Follicle size is larger and contains more oil

____ Objective of a facial is to stimulate oil production for protection of the skin surface

____ Has a good water-oil balance

____ Characterized by gland and pore variation along the T-zone

____ Also known as alipidic skin

a. Dry

b. Normal

c. Oily

d. Combination

86 Where on the face is the T-zone found?

____

____

____

87 List the factors contributing to the formation of wrinkles.

- ____________________
  ____
- ____________________
  ____
- ____________________
  ____
- ____________________
  ____
- ____________________
  ____

Skin Analysis

Fill-in-the-Blank

88 Complete the following guidelines for performing a skin analysis:

1. Observe client's skin ____________, ____________ and appearance; feel the ____________.
2. Ask the client questions relating to the skin's ____________ and ____________ routine.
3. Discuss the facial procedure and/or ____________ plans as well as the ____________ that will be used and why.
4. Encourage the client to ask questions and then determine a ____________ together.
5. ____________ for the client's next visit.

Skin Care Products

Fill-in-the-Blank/Matching

89 Products designed for skin care can usually be categorized as ____________, ____________, ____________, ____________ and ____________

90 Products should be removed from their containers with ____________.

91 Match the correct skin care product with each description.

_____ May contain up to 35 percent alcohol and may be used for oily and acne-prone skin

_____ Water-based products with neutral or slightly acidic pH effective on oily and combination skin types

_____ Formulated to add moisture to the skin surface

_____ Designed to tone or tighten the skin and maybe used on normal and combination skin types

_____ Usually contain 0 to 4 percent alcohol and are suitable for dry, mature, and sensitive skin

_____ Heavier oil-based emulsions that are used primarily to dissolve dirt and makeup

a. Cleansing creams

b. Toners

c. Fresheners

d. Face washes

e. Moisturizers

f. Astringents

92 Witch hazel works as an ____________________ and can be used as a ____________________ tonic in facial treatments and ____________________ services.

93 ____________________ are products that help to physically remove ____________________ from the skin surface and to clear clogged ____________________.

94 Rolling cream is a thick, smooth, ____________________ exfoliating cream.

95 Rolling cream is not recommended on ____________________, ____________________, ____________________, or ____________________ skin.

96 ____________________ loosen or dissolve dead-cell ____________________ on the skin ____________________.

97 ____________________ help to draw impurities out of the ____________________; they can ____________________, ____________________, ____________________, ____________________, and ____________________ the skin.

98 A mask is usually a ____________________, which means that it ____________________ after application.

99 Match the correct mask type with each description.

_____ Are used to stimulate circulation and temporarily contract the skin pores

_____ Often contain humectants and emollients and have a strong moisturizing effect

_____ Use hydrators and smoothing ingredients to add moisture to sensitive and dehydrated skin for a more supple appearance.

_____ Employ the pack application method.

a. Gel

b. Paraffin wax

c. Cream

d. Clay

100 Massage creams are ______________________, ______________________, or ______________________ that provide ______________________ during massage.

101 List the steps in which skin care products are generally used in order from 1 to 8. The first has been filled in for you.

_____ Freshener (low alcohol content)

_____ Moisturizer

_____ Massage cream

_____ Exfoliant (scrub or rolling cream)

_____ Toner or astringent

__1__ Cleansing cream or lotion

_____ Mask or pack

_____ Cleansing cream or lotion

A Note About Men's Skin Care Products

Fill-in-the-Blank

102 Some men do not like ______________________ or ______________________ products.

103 Men seem to prefer ______________________ routines and ______________________ products.

Identify Different Facial Treatments

Fill-in-the-Blank

104 As a professional barber, you should be able to provide different facial ______________________ and ______________________ for different skin ______________________.

Basic Facial

Fill-in-the-Blank

105 The basic facial is sometimes known as the ______________________ facial.

106 A basic facial includes ______________________, ______________________, ______________________, ______________________, a ______________________ or ______________________, and ______________________.

Facial Massage Manipulations

Short Answer/Case Study

107 List the materials, implements, and equipment necessary to perform facial massage manipulations:

- ______________________________
- ______________________________
- ______________________________
- ______________________________
- ______________________________
- ______________________________
- ______________________________
- ______________________________
- ______________________________
- ______________________________
- ______________________________
- ______________________________

108 Rolling Cream Facials IRL

Search for a "rolling cream facial" video online. Watch the video carefully and take note of the way it is performed. How does it differ from the basic facial covered in this chapter? The reality is that many real-world services have their own twist on the basic version of a facial. Describe in your own words how a basic rolling cream facial can be upgraded and still meet the basic requirements of a facial.

____
____
____
____
____
____
____
____
____
____

Vibratory Facial

Fill-in-the-Blank

109 A vibratory facial is often performed using a combination of ______________________ and an ______________________.

110 ______________________ is performed by attaching the massager to your ______________________ and allowing the vibrations to travel through your fingertips or palms to the client's skin.

111 ______________________ requires that you place your ______________________ palm or fingertips on the client's skin with the hand holding the massager on top of your hand.

112 Indirect application is more suitable for ______________________ areas, such as those around the ______________________ and ______________________.

Facial for Dry Skin

Multiple Choice

113 The objective of a facial for dry skin is to help ______________________ the face.

a. moisturize

b. exfoliate

c. relax

d. stimulate

114 Dry skin facials can be supplemented with:

a. ultraviolet rays.

b. rolling cream.

c. high-frequency current.

d. astringents.

Facial for Oily Skin

Fill-in-the-Blank

115 Oily skin and/or ______________________ are caused by hardened masses of ______________________ formed inside a follicle.

116 ______________________ is a disorder of the sebaceous glands.

117 Barbers should wear ______________________ and use only ______________________ movements to apply gentle massage or products to avoid spreading ______________________ matter to other areas of the client's skin.

118 With a treatment plan prescribed by a physician, barbers are limited to performing the following related procedures:

- Reduction of ______________________ on the skin through ______________________ applications
- Removal of ______________________ using proper procedures
- Application of ______________________ or prescribed ______________________

Guidelines for Facial Treatments

Short Answer

119 List five guidelines that will ensure successful facial treatments that can result in repeat booking and referrals.

- ____
  ____
  ____
- ____
  ____
  ____
- ____
  ____
  ____
- ____
  ____
  ____
- ____
  ____
  ____

Word Review

Fill-in-the-Blank

Complete the definitions.

Anaphoresis: The use of the negative pole (cathode) to force an alkaline-pH product, such as a ____________________ lotion, into the skin

Astringent: Tonic lotions with an alcohol content of up to ____________________; used to remove oil accumulation on oily and acne-prone skin.

Cataphoresis: The use of the ____________________ (anode) to introduce an acid-pH product, such as an astringent solution, into the skin.

Contraindication: Any product, procedure, or treatment that should be avoided because it may cause undesirable ____________________ or be ____________________ to the individual.

Direct surface application: ____________________ current performed with the mushroom- or ____________________ electrodes for its calming and germicidal effect on the skin.

Effleurage: Light, continuous ____________________ applied with the fingers (digital) or the palms (palmar) in a slow, rhythmic manner.

Electric massager: Massaging unit that attaches to the barber's hand to impart ______________ massage ______________ to the skin surface.

Friction: Deep rubbing movement requiring ______________ on the skin with the fingers or palm while moving the hand over an underlying structure.

Indirect application: High-frequency current administered with the client holding the wire glass ______________ between both hands.

Iontophoresis: The process of using galvanic current to enable ______________ water-soluble solutions to penetrate the skin.

Microcurrent: Type of ______________ that uses a very low level of electrical current for different applications in skin care.

Microdermabrasion: A form of mechanical ______________ that involves spraying aluminum oxide or other microcrystals across the skin's surface to ______________ dead cells.

Motor point: Point on the skin, over a muscle, where pressure or stimulation will cause ______________ of that muscle.

Percussion: Another name for ______________.

Pétrissage: ______________ movement performed by lifting, squeezing, and pressing the tissue with a light, firm pressure.

Rolling cream: Cleansing and exfoliating product used in ______________ to lift dead skin cells and dirt from the skin surface.

Skin tonics: Toners, fresheners, and astringents; products used to help rebalance skin ______________, remove product residue, and create a temporary ______________ on the skin

Tapotement: Most stimulating massage movement, consisting of short, quick ______________ and ______________ movements.

Trigger point: A tender area in a muscle caused by a ______________ or spasm in the muscle fiber that can radiate pain to other locations in the body.

Vibration: In massage, the ______________ of the body part while the fingertips are pressed firmly on the point of application.

LEARNING OBJECTIVES

After completing this chapter, you will be able to:

- **LO1 List basic guidelines for shaving a client.**
- **LO2 Identify the 14 shaving areas of the face.**
- **LO3 Explain what you need to know about razor positions and strokes to perform a shave safely and effectively.**
- **LO4 Describe the differences between various facial hair designs.**
- **LO5 Discuss Infection Control and safety precautions associated with shaving.**
- **LO6 Demonstrate how to handle a straight razor safely.**
- **LO7 Demonstrate the freehand, backhand, reverse-freehand,and reverse-backhand positions and strokes.**
- **LO8 Demonstrate a shave service.**
- **LO9 Demonstrate a neck shave.**
- **LO10 Demonstrate a mustache trim.**
- **LO11 Demonstrate cutting in beard designs.**

Introduction

Short Answer/Fill-in-the-Blank

1 In your opinion, what are the benefits for men to have a professional shave over shaving at home?

____

____

____

____

____

____

____

____

2 When performed correctly, a full facial shave, complete with ____________________, ____________________, and ____________________, is one of the most relaxing, yet rejuvenating, services men can enjoy in the barbershop.

Why Study Shaving and Facial-Hair Design?

3 List two reasons studying shaving and facial-hair design is important for a barber.

1. ____
____
____

2. ____
____
____

Understand the Fundamentals of Shaving

LO 1 **List basic guidelines for shaving a client.**

LO 2 **Identify the 14 shaving areas of the face.**

LO 3 **Explain what you need to know about razor positions and strokes to perform a shave safely and effectively.**

Consider Basic Guidelines for Shaving a Client

Fill-in-the-Blank/Case Study

4 Do not proceed with the service if the client has a ____________________ or ____________________.

5 ____________________ the client's hair growth pattern before beginning the shave to identify grain changes and growth patterns in the beard.

6 Do not use ____________________ on skin that is chapped, blistered, thin, or sensitive.

7 Do not perform a(n) ____________________ immediately after a shave as it may irritate or damage the skin.

8 Use ____________________ fresheners or ____________________ when stronger astringents are too harsh for sensitive skin.

9 When a client wears a ____________________, trim and shape it prior to the shave service to prepare it for finish work with the razor during the shave.

10 Be careful when shaving sensitive areas beneath the ____________________, on the lower part of the ____________________, and around the Adam's apple to avoid irritation or injury.

11 Knowing When Not to Shave

A shave service has many benefits for the client, such as relaxation. However, there are times when a client must be declined for a shave service. Identify one or two instances in which you would have to tell a client that a shave cannot be performed and explain why. Explain what you would do instead.

____

____

____

____

____

____

____

____

Identifying the Shaving Areas of the Face

Labeling

12 Number the shaving areas in the following illustration depending on whether you are right-handed or left-handed. Next, draw the directional arrows for each area.

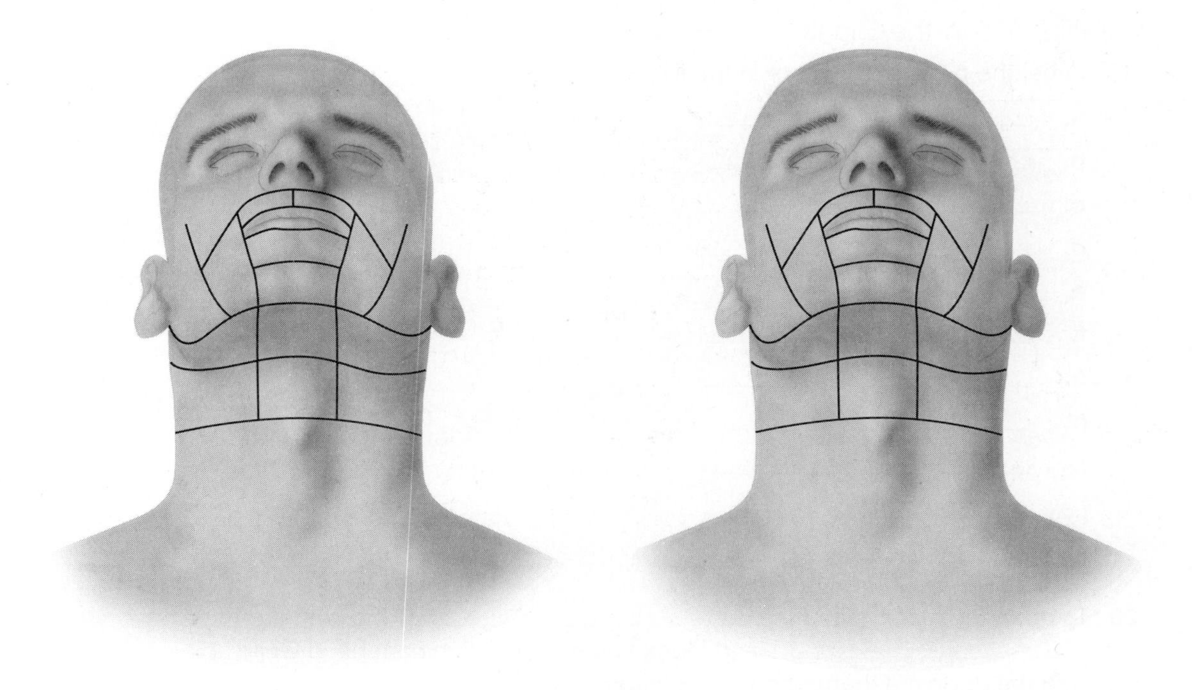

Understand Razor Positions and Strokes

Fill-in-the-Blank

13 To achieve a proper cutting stroke, the razor is positioned at a slight __________ to the skin surface and stroked with the point __________.

14 The three positions and strokes used in facial shaving are __________, __________, and __________.

15 __________ refers to the way the razor is held in the barber's hand to perform a stroke movement.

16 It is important to know how to position the fingers, wrist, and elbow of the __________ hand in relation to the razor.

17 A barber must know how to use the __________ and __________ finger as the primary digits for stretching the skin.

18 A barber must angle the razor about __________ degrees relative to the skin surface.

Handling a Straight Razor (Procedure 13-1)

LO 6 **Demonstrate how to handle a straight razor safely.**

Labeling/Fill-in-the-Blank

19 Label the parts of the razor in the illustration.

a. __________

b. __________

c. __________

d. __________

e. __________

f. __________

g. __________

h. __________

i. __________

j. __________

k. __________

20 To open the razor, grasp the __________ of the blade between the __________ and index finger of the dominant hand while holding the handle with the opposite thumb and index finger.

21 Hold the razor between the thumb and index finger on the sides of the __________ near the shoulder of the blade and rest across the __________ and third fingers, with the __________ finger bracing the razor.

22 When closing the razor, release the __________ finger and bring the __________ to the blade.

Razor Position and Strokes Practice (Procedure 13-2)

LO 7 **Demonstrate the freehand, backhand, reverse-freehand, and reverse-backhand positions and strokes.**

Matching/Short Answer/Fill-in-the-Blank

23 Match the descriptions with the correct razor position and stroke.

_____ Handle of razor should rest between the third and fourth fingers

_____ Underside of handle rests on the third and fourth fingers

_____ Left hand should be positioned above the razor

_____ Razor edge should be turned upward

a. Freehand

b. Backhand

c. Reverse-freehand

d. Reverse-backhand

24 List the shaving areas in which the freehand position and stroke is used.

- ______________________________
- ______________________________
- ______________________________
- ______________________________
- ______________________________
- ______________________________

25 Explain when the reverse backhand stroke may be used.

____

____

26 List the shaving areas in which the backhand stroke is used.

- ______________________________
- ______________________________
- ______________________________
- ______________________________
- ______________________________

27 With the reverse-backhand position and stroke, use a smooth, ______________ stroke, directed ______________ that leads with the point of the razor.

28 With the reverse-freehand position and stroke, use a(n) ______________, semi-arced stroke toward you with the point leading in a ______________ movement.

29 With the freehand stroke, ______________ with the point of the razor in a ______________, gliding movement.

Understand Body Positioning

Fill-in-the-Blank

30 If you are a right-handed barber, you will stand at the client's ______________________ side.

31 If you are a left-handed barber, you will stand at the client's ______________________ side.

32 To change position, take ______________________ steps or shift your body weight from one ______________________ to the other.

Describe the Professional Shave

Multiple Choice

33 The skin is held ______________________ to create the correct shaving surface for the razor.

a. tightly

b. loosely

c. firmly

d. not at all

34 When shaving a client, excess lather should be removed with the ______________________

a. thumb

b. forefinger

c. index finger

d. pinky finger

35 ______________________ skin allows the beard hair to be cut more easily.

a. Dry

b. Loose

c. Bumpy

d. Taut

Know the Types of Shaves

Fill-in-the-Blank/Short Answer/Multiple Choice

36 A(n) ______________________ shave should ensure a complete and even shave with a single lathering.

37 ______________________ is the practice of shaving the beard against the grain during the second-time-over phase of the shave.

38 With the second-time-over shave, the client's skin is moistened with a(n) ______________________ towel or water and a(n) ______________________ stroke is used to shave with or across the grain to remove any remaining hair.

39 Describe the difference between a traditional neck shave and an outline shave.

____

____

____

____

____

____

____

40 Which part of the head and neck is *not* shaved during a traditional neck shave?

a. Behind the ears.
b. Across the nape.
c. Both sides of the neck.
d. Front hairline.

Understand Facial-Hair Design: Mustaches

LO 4 **Describe the differences between various facial hair designs.**

Multiple Choice/Matching

41 Which of the following characteristics of facial features does *not* influence mustache design?

a. Size of the nose.
b. Shape of upper lip area.
c. Size of the eyes.
d. Width of the mouth.

42 Match the facial features with the appropriate mustache design.

_____ Long, narrow face
_____ Extra-small mouth
_____ Round face with regular features
_____ Square face with prominent features
_____ Extra-large mouth
_____ Prominent nose
_____ Large, coarse facial features
_____ Wide mouth with prominent upper lip
_____ Smallish, regular features

a. Heavier-looking mustache
b. Medium to large mustache
c. Narrow to medium mustache
d. Pyramid-shaped mustache
e. Medium, short mustache
f. Smaller, triangular mustache
g. Heavier handlebar or large divided mustache
h. Semi-square mustache
i. Heavier, linear mustache with ends slightly curving downward

Designing the Beard

Fill-in-the-Blank

43 Analyze the ______________________ and ______________________ of the hair to identify uneven growth areas.

44 Consider where hair growth under the ______________________ and ______________________ changes direction to help determine design options for outlines in this area.

45 Leave the facial hair slightly ______________________ than the desired end result during the ______________________ trimming to avoid cutting the hair too closely.

46 ______________________ clipper-cutting is most successful on beards with even density and texture.

47 Beard trimming and design is usually performed with a combination of the ______________________, ______________________, outliner and/or clippers, and razor.

Review Shaving-Related Infection Control and Safety Precautions

LO 5 **Discuss infection control and safety precautions associated with shaving.**

Fill-in-the-Blank

48 ______________________ and ______________________ razors and blades before use.

49 ______________________ used blades in a sharps container.

50 Wash your hands ______________________ servicing a client.

51 Use ______________________ linens, capes, and paper products.

52 Provide a clean cloth or paper barrier between the client's head and the ______________________.

53 Treat small cuts or nicks using standard precautions and ______________________ procedures.

54 ______________________ the chair once the client is properly draped and in position for the shave.

55 Prepare ______________________ hair for the shave with warm or hot towels and lather.

56 Use a light touch and a forward ______________________ motion that leads with the point of the blade.

57 Observe the ______________________ and shave with it, not against it.

58 ______________________ against the grain gently to place the hair in a position to be shaved.

59 Keep your fingers ______________________ to stretch or hold the skin firmly during the shave.

60 Use the cushions of the fingertips to stretch skin in the ______________________ direction of the razor stroke.

61 Keep the fingers and thumb of the ______________________ hand away from the path of the razor.

62 Apply ______________________ neatly to the areas to be shaved and replace as necessary.

63 Keep the skin ______________________ while shaving.

64 Follow through with shaving strokes from one shaving area to another; do not stop ______________________ or shave over an area repeatedly.

Word Review

Fill-in-the-Blank

Backhand	Neck shave	Second-time-over shave
Cutting stroke	Once-over shave	Styptic powder
First-time-over shave	Reverse backhand	
Freehand	Reverse freehand	

______________________: Alum powder or liquid used to stop bleeding of nicks and cuts.

______________________: Razor position and stroke used in 4 of the 14 basic shaving areas: nos. 2, 6, 7, and 9; optional position for area 12.

______________________: A single-lather shave in which the shaving strokes are made across the grain of the hair.

______________________: A razor position and stroke used in 4 of the 14 basic shaving areas: nos. 5, 10, 13, and 14.

______________________: The first part of the standard shave consisting of shaving the 14 areas of the face; followed by the second-time-over shave to remove residual missed or rough spots.

______________________: A shaving technique that follows a regular shave to remove any rough or uneven spots using water instead of lather; may be considered a form of close shaving.

______________________: Razor position and stroke used in 6 of the 14 shaving areas: nos. 1, 3, 4, 8, 11, and 12.

______________________: The correct angle of cutting the beard with a straight razor.

______________________: Shaving the areas behind the ears down the sides of the neck, and at the back neckline.

______________________: A razor position and stroke used by right-handed barbers for shaving the left side of the neck behind the ear and used by left-handed barbers behind the right ear.

CHAPTER 14 MEN'S HAIRCUTTING AND STYLING

LEARNING OBJECTIVES

After completing this chapter, you will be able to:

LO1 Explain the importance of the client consultation and consider questions that help you envision the client's desired outcome.

LO2 Describe anatomical features that influence haircutting and styling.

LO3 Identify the sections of the head as applied to haircutting.

LO4 Identify tapering and blending areas.

LO5 Define design elements used in haircutting and styling.

LO6 Define basic terms used in haircutting and styling.

LO7 Explain basic cutting techniques using shears, clippers, and razors.

LO8 Describe basic haircut styles.

LO9 Describe haircut finish work.

LO10 Describe basic styling techniques.

LO11 Discuss haircutting and styling safety precautions.

LO12 Demonstrate basic haircuts and styling techniques.

Introduction

Short Answer/Fill-in-the-Blank

1 List three reasons why studying and having a good understanding of men's haircutting and styling is important for barbers.

a. ______________________________

____

____

b. ______________________________

____

____

c. ______________________________

____

____

2 The term *styling* usually refers to ______________, ______________, ______________, or other methods used to ______________ or ______________ the hair into its finished look.

3 Haircutting and styling requires that the barber consider the client's head ______________, ______________, ______________ length, ______________, and hair ______________.

Why Study Men's Haircutting and Styling?

Multiple Choice

4 Barbers should have a thorough understanding of men's haircutting and styling because:

a. They will know what treatment products to use.

b. They will know when to replace equipment.

c. It is the foundation of the profession.

d. They can enter competitions and win.

Understand the Importance of the Client Consultation

LO 1 **Explain the importance of the client consultation and consider questions that help you envision the client's desired outcome.**

Fill-in-the-Blank

5 The client consultation is a ______________ between you and the client about the client's ______________ and ______________ of the service you will perform.

6 During a consultation, it is important to identify ______________, such as ______________, ______________, or ______________, that may limit or enhance cutting and styling options.

7 During a consultation, the barber should discover ______________ that may prohibit moving forward with the service.

Discuss Common Questions Asked During a Consultation

Short Answer

8 Identify four basic questions that should be asked during a client consultation.

1. ______________________________

2. ______________________________

3. ______________________________

4. ______________________________

9 What is the best way to avoid any confusion or pricing issues due to misinterpretations of what a *trim* means?

____

____

____

Know Basic Principles of Haircutting and Styling

LO 2 Describe anatomical features that influence haircutting and styling.

LO 3 Identify the sections of the head as applied to haircutting.

LO 4 Identify tapering and blending areas.

LO 5 Define design elements used in haircutting and styling.

LO 6 Define basic terms used in haircutting and styling.

Recognize Anatomical Features

Facial Shapes

Fill-in-the-Blank/Matching

10 Describe the shapes of the faces in the images below.

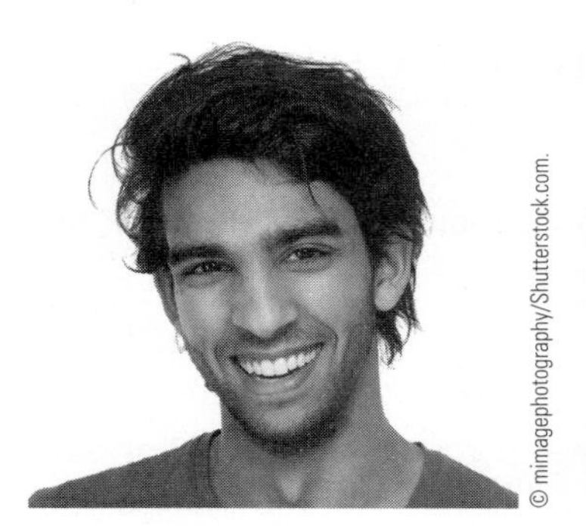

© mimagephotography/Shutterstock.com.

____

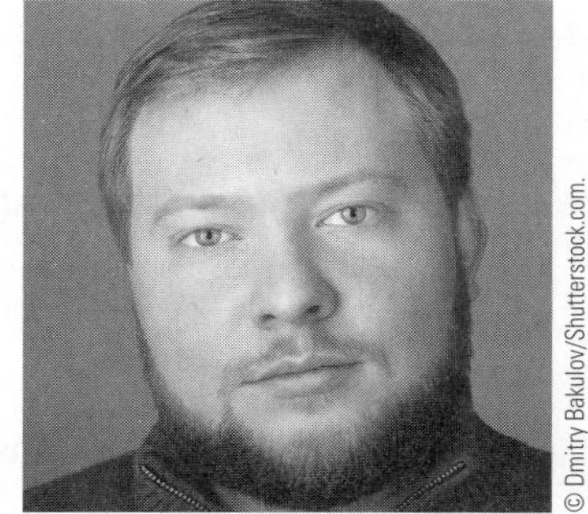

© Dmitry Bakulov/Shutterstock.com.

____

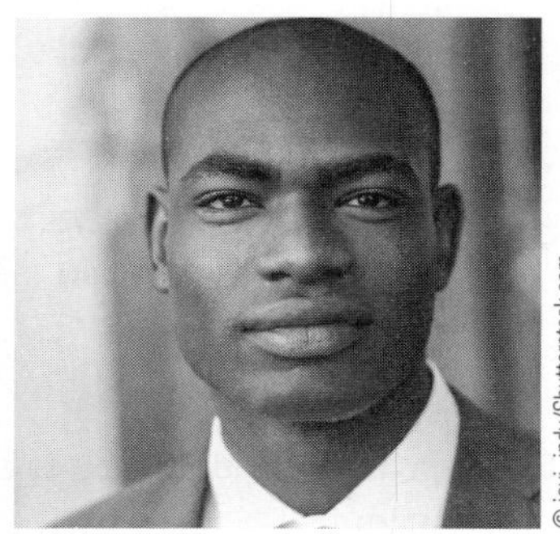

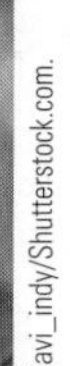

© javi_indy/Shutterstock.com.

____

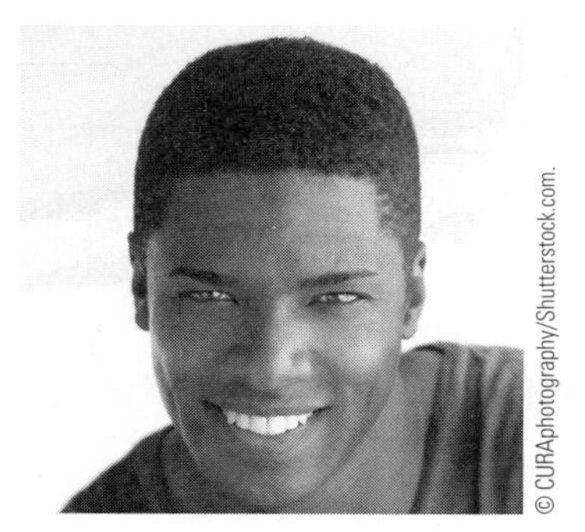

© CURAphotography/Shutterstock.com.

____

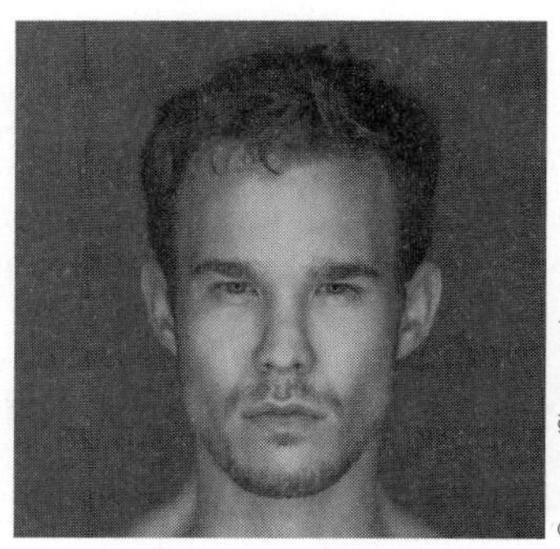

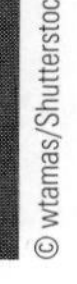

© wtamas/Shutterstock.com.

____

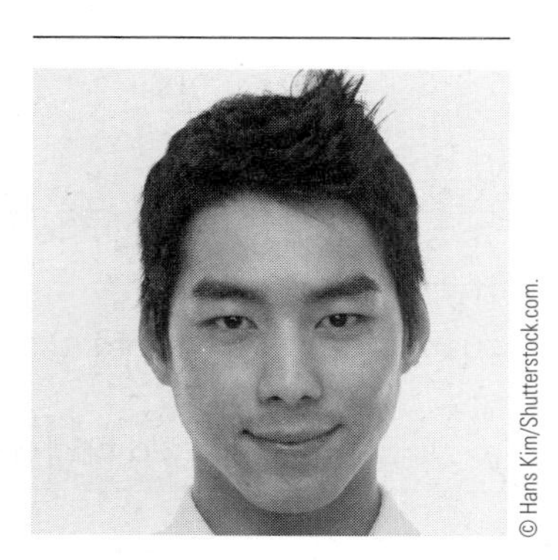

© Hans Kim/Shutterstock.com.

____

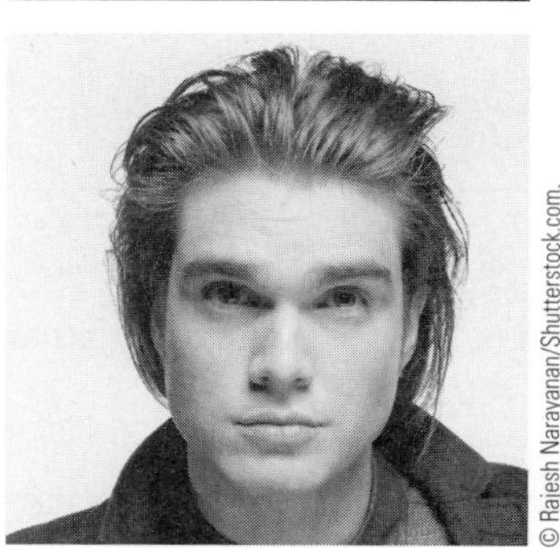

© Rajesh Narayanan/Shutterstock.com.

____

11 Match the haircutting technique with the appropriate facial feature.

_____ Use wavy bangs that blend into the temples to an asymmetrical line

_____ Keep the hair close at the crown and temples and longer in back

_____ Create some height on the top to lengthen the look of the face

_____ Create width and fullness at the top, temples, and sides to produce balance

_____ Layer bangs and brush to the sides over the temples

_____ Keep hair close to the head at the widest points of the face

_____ Change the part or redirect the hair to experiment with different looks

a. Diamond

b. Inverted triangular

c. Oblong

d. Round

e. Square

f. Oval

g. Pear

Head Shapes

Short Answer

12 Give one example of how a client's head shape may not conform to the generalized basic head shape, and how a barber would adapt their haircutting and styling choices in response.

____

____

____

____

____

____

____

____

Profiles

Multiple Choice

13 _________________ profiles have a prominent forehead and chin.

a. Concave
b. Straight
c. Convex
d. Angular

14 _________________ profiles have a receding forehead, but the chin tends to jut forward.

a. Concave
b. Straight
c. Convex
d. Angular

15 _________________ profiles tend to be the most balanced and proportioned because the forehead and chin align with only a slight curvature.

a. Concave
b. Straight
c. Convex
d. Angular

16 ____________ profiles recede at the forehead and chin.

a. Concave
b. Straight
c. Convex
d. Angular

Neck Lengths, Ear Size, and Sideburn Designs

Short Answer

17 What are two guidelines for working with different neck lengths?

- ____

- ____

18 Why is the size and placement of the client's ears important to a haircut design?

____

19 How does a barber determine the most suitable length and shape for a client's sideburns?

____

20 What are two guidelines for designing sideburns?

- ____

- ____

Learn the Sections of the Head Form

Labeling/Fill-in-the-Blank

21 Label the sections of the head in the following figures.

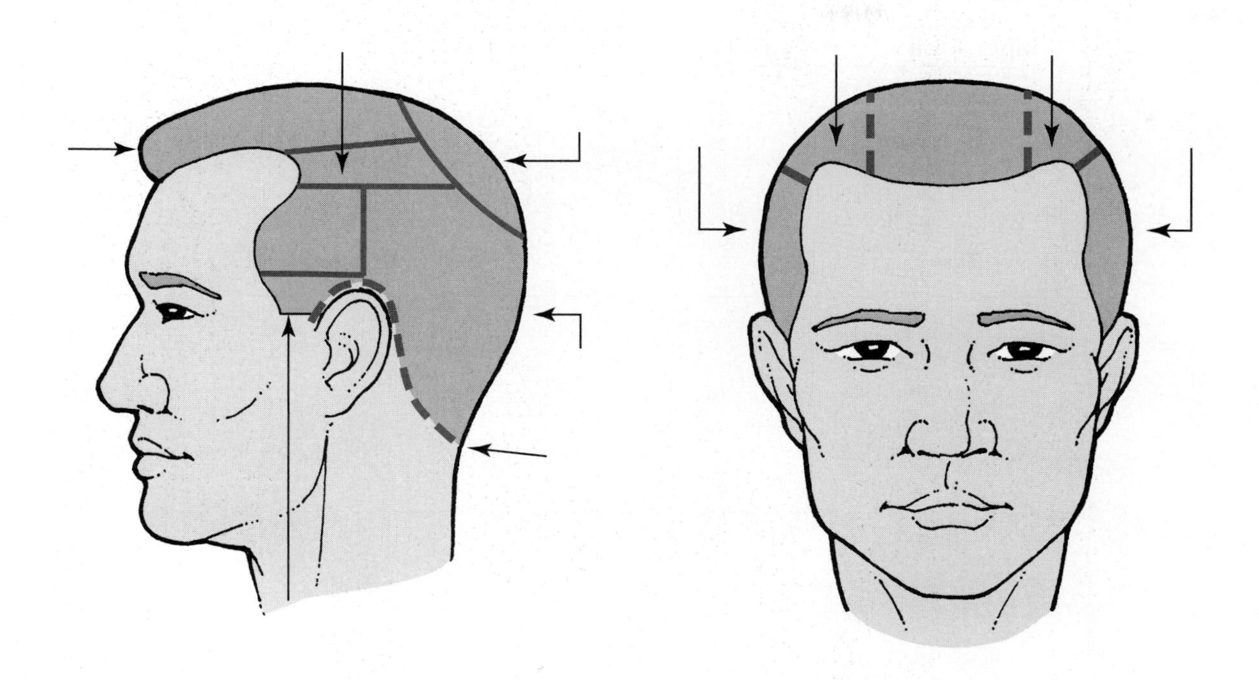

22 ______________________ are points on the head that mark areas where the surface of the head changes or the behavior of the hair changes as a result.

23 The ______________________ is also known as the ______________________, *temporal, horseshoe,* or *hatband* area of the head. It is the ______________________ section of the head.

24 The ______________________ protrudes at the base of the skull. The ______________________ is the highest point on the top of the head. The ______________________ are located by crossing diagonal lines at the ______________________.

Tapering and Blending Areas

Fill-in-the-Blank

24 Identify the appropriate hairstyle (i.e., long, medium, short, semi-short, fade) based on the taper area shown in the images below.

Taper Area	Hairstyle
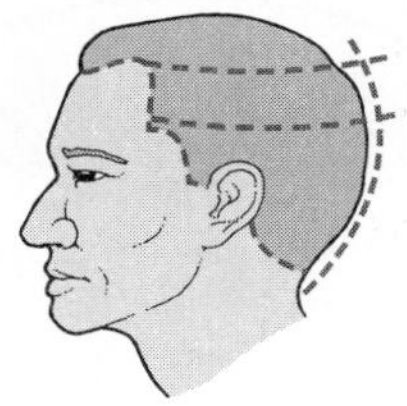	
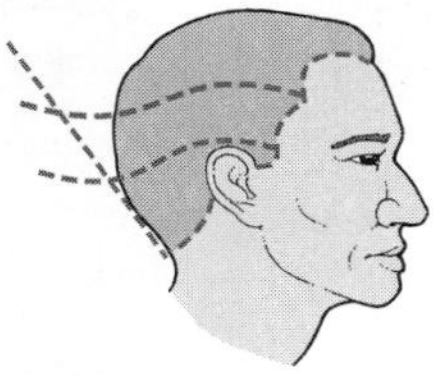	
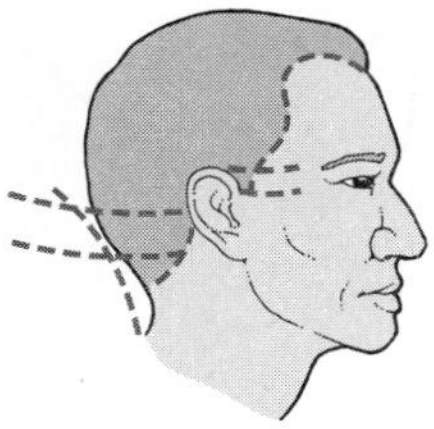	
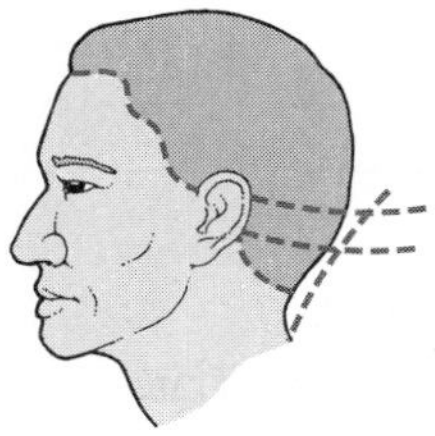	
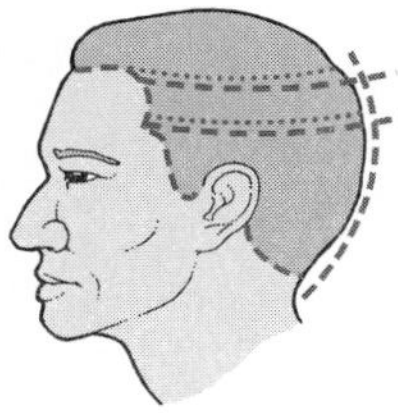	

26 Tapering is the action of gradually ____________ the ____________ of the hair without any lines of demarcation such as ____________ or ____________.

27 Tapering is performed from the ____________ to just below the ____________ and just above the ____________.

28 Medium-length styles do not have a ____________ appearance.

Understand Design Elements Used in Haircutting

Lines

Matching

29 Fill in each statement with the correct type of line from the word bank.

_____	Cutting lines remove weight within the cut and create layers.	**a. Vertical**
_____	Lines have a slanted direction and are used to create sloped lines within a haircut or at the perimeter to determine the design line.	**b. Horizontal**
_____	Lines move in a semicircular or circular direction and can be shallow or deep.	**c. Curved**
_____	Cutting lines build weight and are used to create a one-length look and low elevation or blunt haircuts.	**d. Diagonal**
_____	Lines soften a design; when repeated in opposite directions, they create a wave pattern.	
_____	Lines are parallel to the horizon or floor and direct the eye from one side to the other.	
_____	Finger placement may be used to create a stacked, layered effect at the perimeter.	
_____	Lines are perpendicular to the floor and are described in terms of up and down.	

Form and Space

Fill-in-the-Blank

30 Form is the ______________________ or ______________________ of a hairstyle.

31 ______________________ is the equal or appropriate proportions that create ______________________ and ______________________ in a design.

32 In hair design, the form (haircut or style) occupies ______________________ space and the area that surrounds it is ______________________ space.

Design Texture and Color

Short Answer

33 What does *design texture* refer to? ____.

34 What are some terms used to describe hair texture? ____

____

35 How do different colors act differently in a design? ____

____

Understand Basic Terminology Used in Haircutting and Styling

Angles, Directional Terms, and Cross-checking

Fill-in-the-Blank

36 *Angles* can refer to the ________________________ at which the hair is held for cutting.

37 *Angles* can also refer to the ________________________ when cutting a section of hair.

38 Cutting ________________________ means to cut the hair in the opposite direction from which it grows.

39 Cutting ________________________ means the hair is cut in a direction that is neither with nor against the grain.

40 ________________________ is the process of parting off ________________________ opposite from the elevation or direction at which they were cut to check the ________________________ of cutting lines or ________________________.

Elevation and Projection

Matching/Word Search

41 Match the correct degrees of elevation with each description.

_____ Most common projection used in men's haircutting

_____ Achieved by combing the hair straight down and cutting it against the skin or held straight down

_____ Considered medium elevation

_____ Produces layering, tapering, and blended effects

_____ Used to create a graduated or stacked effect

_____ Used to create layers when cutting long hair

_____ Hair is held straight out from the head from where it grows

_____ Produces weight, bulk, and maximum length at the perimeter of a design

a. 0

b. 45

c. 90

d. 180

42 After determining the correct word from the definition provided, locate the words in the word search.

________________________ The angle or degree at which a section of hair is held from the head for cutting, relative to where it grows.

________________________ A line, created naturally or with a comb, that divides the hair at the scalp, separating one section of the hair from another.

________________________ A smaller section of hair that is parted off from a larger section of hair.

________________________ Established by the angle of the fingers or comb when securing a section of hair for cutting.

________________________ The outer perimeter line of the haircut.

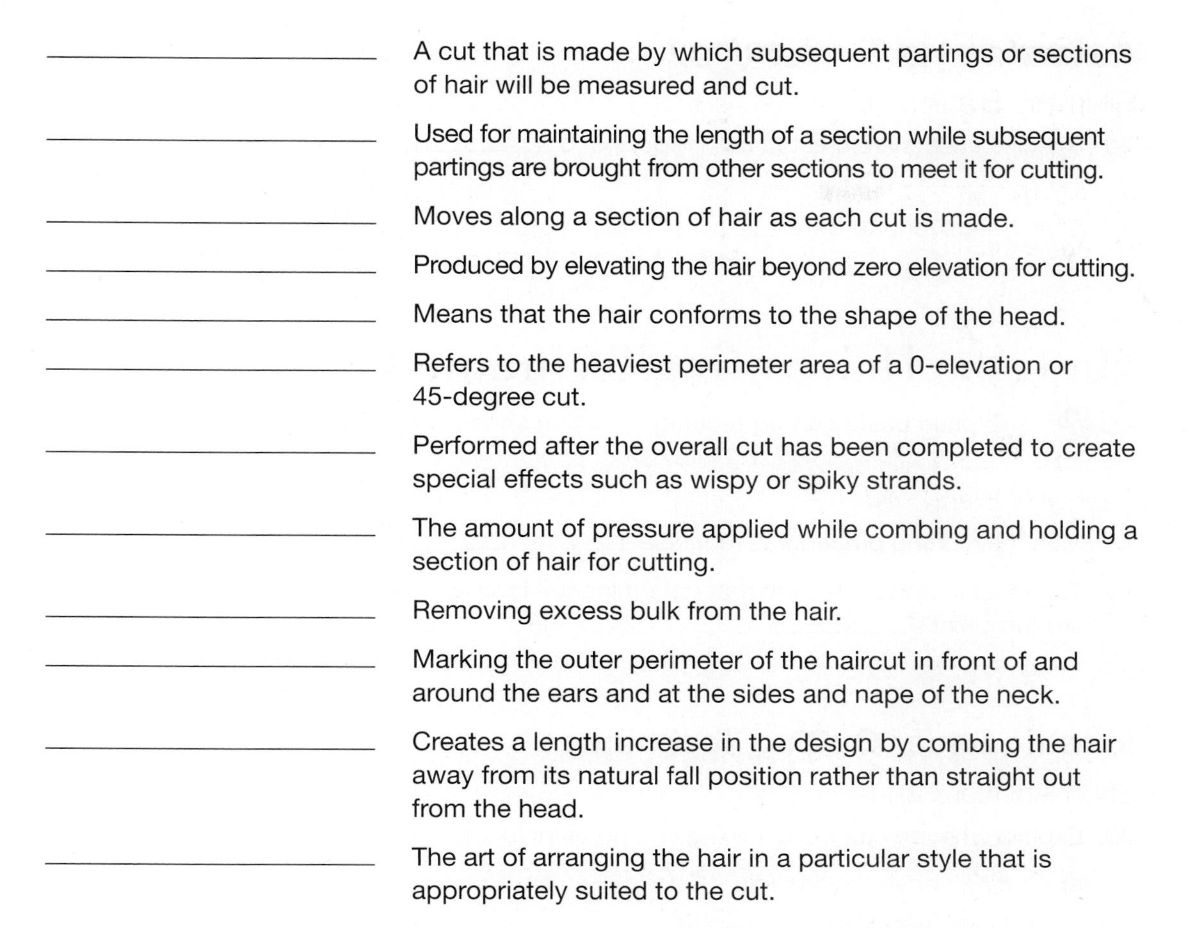

______________________ A cut that is made by which subsequent partings or sections of hair will be measured and cut.

______________________ Used for maintaining the length of a section while subsequent partings are brought from other sections to meet it for cutting.

______________________ Moves along a section of hair as each cut is made.

______________________ Produced by elevating the hair beyond zero elevation for cutting.

______________________ Means that the hair conforms to the shape of the head.

______________________ Refers to the heaviest perimeter area of a 0-elevation or 45-degree cut.

______________________ Performed after the overall cut has been completed to create special effects such as wispy or spiky strands.

______________________ The amount of pressure applied while combing and holding a section of hair for cutting.

______________________ Removing excess bulk from the hair.

______________________ Marking the outer perimeter of the haircut in front of and around the ears and at the sides and nape of the neck.

______________________ Creates a length increase in the design by combing the hair away from its natural fall position rather than straight out from the head.

______________________ The art of arranging the hair in a particular style that is appropriately suited to the cut.

L	H	I	P	P	I	O	Y	C	A	N	L	P	O	R
A	A	I	R	C	U	T	T	I	N	G	L	I	N	E
Y	I	I	C	R	T	N	T	G	N	G	T	I	D	T
E	R	O	V	E	R	D	I	R	E	C	T	I	O	N
R	S	T	E	N	I	A	G	O	T	T	U	T	O	G
S	T	A	T	I	O	N	A	R	Y	G	U	I	D	E
U	Y	P	G	N	G	O	N	U	G	O	S	T	E	E
C	L	E	T	P	U	Z	U	N	L	N	I	H	S	L
P	I	R	G	A	I	L	I	T	E	R	E	T	I	Y
N	N	O	I	R	D	L	N	T	L	G	I	V	G	R
L	G	T	N	T	E	X	T	U	R	I	Z	I	N	G
L	T	N	N	V	T	H	I	N	N	I	N	G	L	I
D	L	P	A	R	T	I	N	G	O	T	I	I	I	I
N	P	R	O	J	E	C	T	I	O	N	Y	T	N	G
T	T	Y	S	W	E	I	G	H	T	L	I	N	E	G

A Word about Terminology

Fill-in-the-Blank

43 Specific effects are created using specific ________________ and ________________.

44 Style trends tend to be ________________ in nature. For example, ________________ were a hit in the 1920s and 1930s.

Describe Haircutting Techniques

LO 7 **Explain basic cutting techniques using shears, clippers, and razors.**

Fill-in-the-Blank

45 Most haircutting procedures require a ________________ of techniques and tools.

46 The most important factors that determine the tools used to achieve the haircut are the client's ________________, the ________________ and ________________ of the hair, and the barber's ________________.

Identify Shear Cutting Techniques

Short Answer/Fill-in-the-Blank

47 Explain when to use the following cutting techniques.

a) Cutting above the fingers:

____

____

____

b) Cutting below the fingers:

____

____

____

c) Shear-over-comb:

____

____

____

d) Freehand shear cutting:

____

____

____

48 The three basic methods for using ________________ are cutting on top of the fingers, cutting below the fingers, and ________________.

49 Shear-over-comb is also used in ______________ to thin out or customize difficult areas caused by hollows, wrinkles, whorls, or creases in the scalp.

Identify Clipper Cutting Techniques

Fill-in-the-Blank

50 Freehand clipper cutting requires a steady hand and consistent use of the ______________ while cutting.

51 True freehand clipper cutting tends to be used on two extremes of hair length: very ______________ straight, ______________, and ______________ lengths; and ______________, ______________ curled hair lengths.

52 The freehand method is also used to ______________ hairlines at the ______________, ______________, and ______________.

53 The use of ______________ is not usually acceptable for state board practical examinations.

54 ______________ cutting can be used for the entire haircut or to ______________ the hair from shorter tapered areas to longer areas at the top, crest, or occipital.

Razor Cutting

Matching/Fill-in-the-Blank

55 Fill in each statement with the correct razor cutting technique from the word bank.

_____ is performed by holding the hair section between your fingers and cutting either from the top to the bottom of the section or from one side to the other.

_____ is performed by using a rotating motion with the comb and razor as the hair is being cut.

_____ can be performed in two different ways using a freehand razor position.

_____ is also known as *freehand slicing*.

a. Razor-over-comb cutting

b. Razor rotation

c. Fingers-and-razor cutting

56 Fill in each statement with the correct taper-blending method from the word bank.

In _____, the angle of the razor blade is increased to almost 90 degrees, producing the least amount of tapering to the hair ends.

_____ is performed with the razor held up to 45 degrees from the surface of the hair strand, increasing the depth of the cut as the angle and pressure increases.

In _____, the razor is held almost flat against the surface of the hair, cutting only a small amount of hair using very little pressure.

a. light taper-blending

b. heavier taper-blending

c. terminal blending

57 When razor cutting fine hair, use a ______________ strike of the razor with ______________ pressure.

58 The hair must be ______________ and ______________ for best results and to avoid client discomfort.

59 Handle the razor properly, keeping it ______________ whenever not in use.

60 Hair ______________ is used to reduce the bulk or weight of the hair.

61 Three methods that can be used to reduce bulky or thick areas within a hair design are ______________, ______________, and ______________.

62 ______________ or ______________ with regular shears can be used to reduce weight in the ends of the hair.

Recognize Basic Haircut Styles

LO 8 **Describe basic haircut styles.**

Fill-in-the-Blank

63 Identify the type of haircut in the images below.

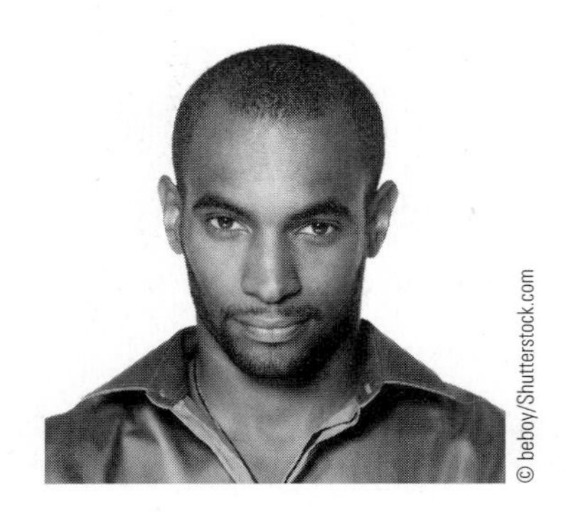

____

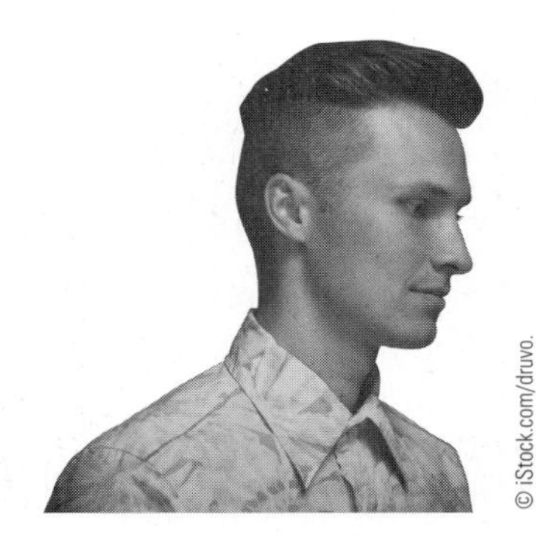

____

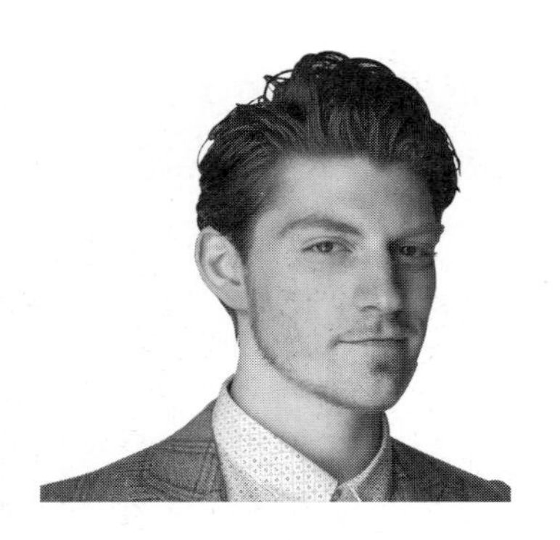

____

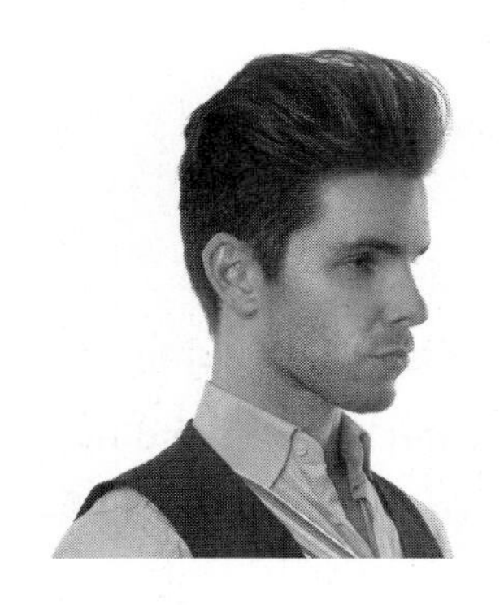

____

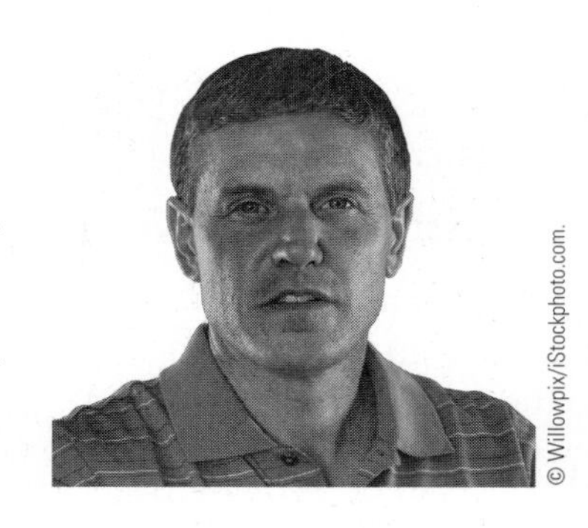

____

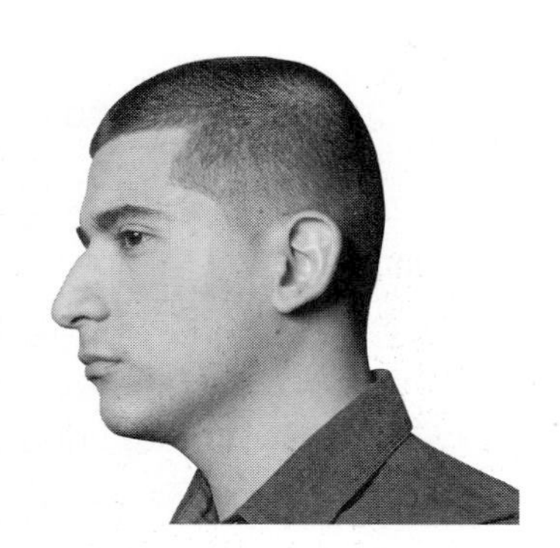

____

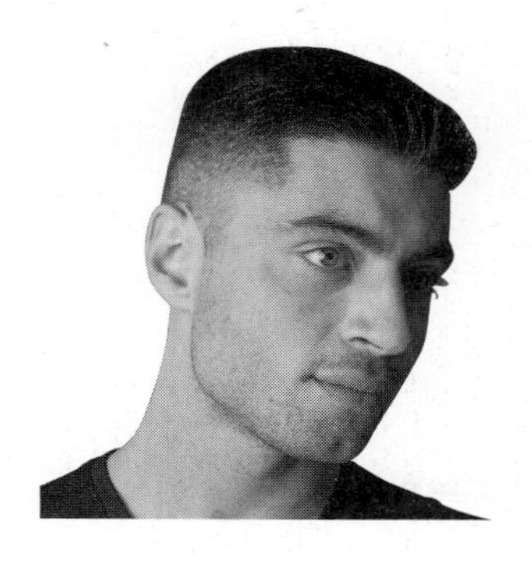

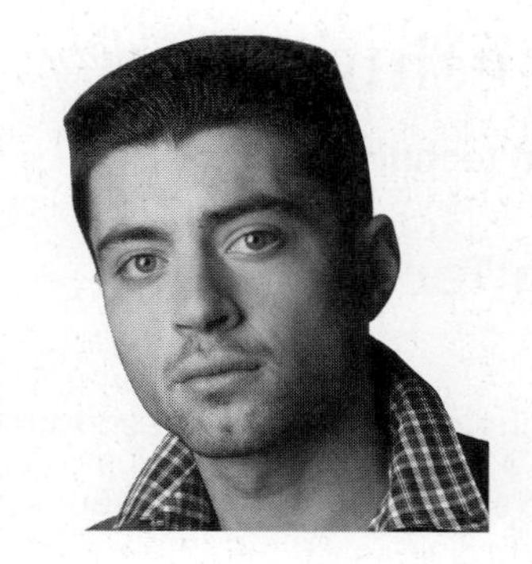

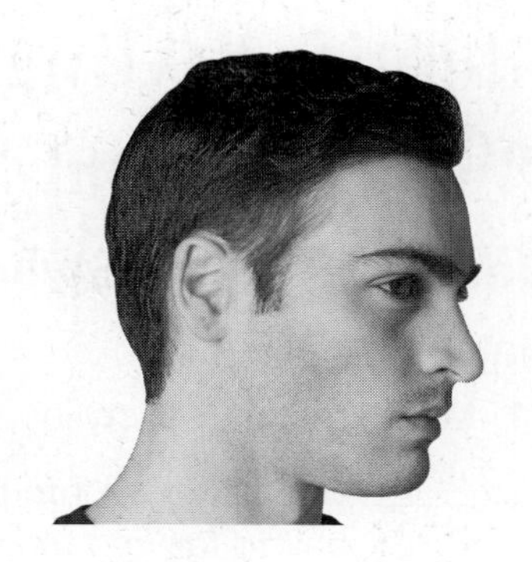

______________________ ______________________ ______________________

Explain Haircut Finish Work

LO 9 **Describe haircut finish work.**

Shaving and Trimming

Fill-in-the-Blank

64 The traditional ______________________ consists of shaving the sides of the neck and across the nape with a razor.

65 The ______________________ starts at the bottom of the sideburns, arches around and behind the ears, down the sides of the neck, and across the nape.

66 The ______________________ technique is the most popular technique for eyebrow trimming.

67 Safety and protection of the client's ______________________ should always be the first consideration when using any eyebrow-trimming technique.

68 Outliners with ______________________ blades or ______________________ are the safest tools to use for trimming excess hair from the nostrils.

69 To shave a head, the hair and scalp are prepared with ______________________ and lather followed by ______________________ shaving.

70 When beginning a head shave, thoroughly ______________________ the scalp to identify moles and other ______________________.

Identify Styling Techniques

LO 10 Describe basic styling techniques.

Describe Basic Styling Techniques

Matching

71 Match the correct styling technique with each description.

_____ Build fullness into the style whileallowing the hair to fall into the natural lines of cut

_____ Shape and direct hair into an S pattern using the fingers, comb, and styling lotion

_____ Dry and style damp hair in one operation

_____ Use a diffuser attachment while lifting and squeezing the hair with the fingers

_____ Use the fingers to manipulate the hair into place instead of a comb or brush

_____ Leave the hair to air-dry naturally

_____ Maintain the natural wave pattern of the hair, as opposed to temporarily straightening it

_____ Dry each section of hair in a definite direction with the aid of a comb or brush with dryer

a. Natural drying

b. Finger styling

c. Scrunch styling

d. Finger waving

e. Blowdry styling

f. Freeform blowdrying

g. Stylized blowdrying

h. Diffused drying

Braids and Locks

Fill-in-the-Blank

72 ____________________ require working close to the scalp across the curves of the head.

73 ____________________ is the process that occurs when coiled hair is allowed to develop in its natural state.

74 ____________________ are those that are intentionally guided through the natural process of locking.

75 Two basic methods for locking men's hair are the ____________________ and the ____________________ method.

Discuss Safety Precautions for Haircutting and Styling

LO 11 Discuss haircutting and styling safety precautions.

Case Study

76 Safety Precautions

Barbers must be aware of the hazards that exist in the barbershop while cutting and styling a client's hair. Barbers must take the safety precautions mentioned in this chapter, however many barbers take additional precautions. Identify additional safety precautions you would take that are not mentioned in this chapter and explain why you would take such measures.

____

____

____

____

____

____

____

____

____

____

Word Review

Crossword Puzzle

Find the correct term in the crossword puzzle using the clues provided.

Across

Clue

3. The angle or degree at which a subsection of hair is held, or elevated, from the head when cutting; also referred to as projection.
4. The section of hair, located at either the perimeter or the interior of the cut, that determines the length the hair will be cut to; also referred to as a guideline; usually the first section that is cut to create a shape.
6. A visual line in the haircut, where the ends of the hair hang together; the line of maximum length within the weight area: heaviest perimeter area of a 0-degree (one-length) or 45-degree (graduated) cut.

Down

Clue

1. The process that occurs when coiled hair is allowed to develop in its natural state without the use of combs, heat, or chemicals.
2. Oval, round, inverted triangular, square, oblong, diamond, and pear-shaped are the seven facial shapes.
5. Lines that are straight up and down.
8. Combing a section away from its natural falling position, rather than straight out from the head, toward a guideline; used to create increasing lengths in the interior or perimeter.

Across

Clue

7. The space between two lines or surfaces that intersect at a given point; in haircutting, the hair is held away from the head to create an angle of elevation.
11. A texturizing technique similar to razor-over-comb, done with small circular motions.
12. A graduated effect achieved by cutting the hair with elevation or over-direction; the hair is cut at higher elevations, usually 90 degrees or above, which removes weight.
13. The equal or appropriate proportions that create symmetry and harmony in a design.
14. The widest area of the head, also known as the parietal ridge, temporal region, hatband, or horseshoe.
15. A guideline that does not move, but all other hair is brought to it for cutting.

Down

Clue

9. The widest area of the head, also known as the crest, hatband, horseshoe, or temporal region.
10. Usually the perimeter line of a haircut.

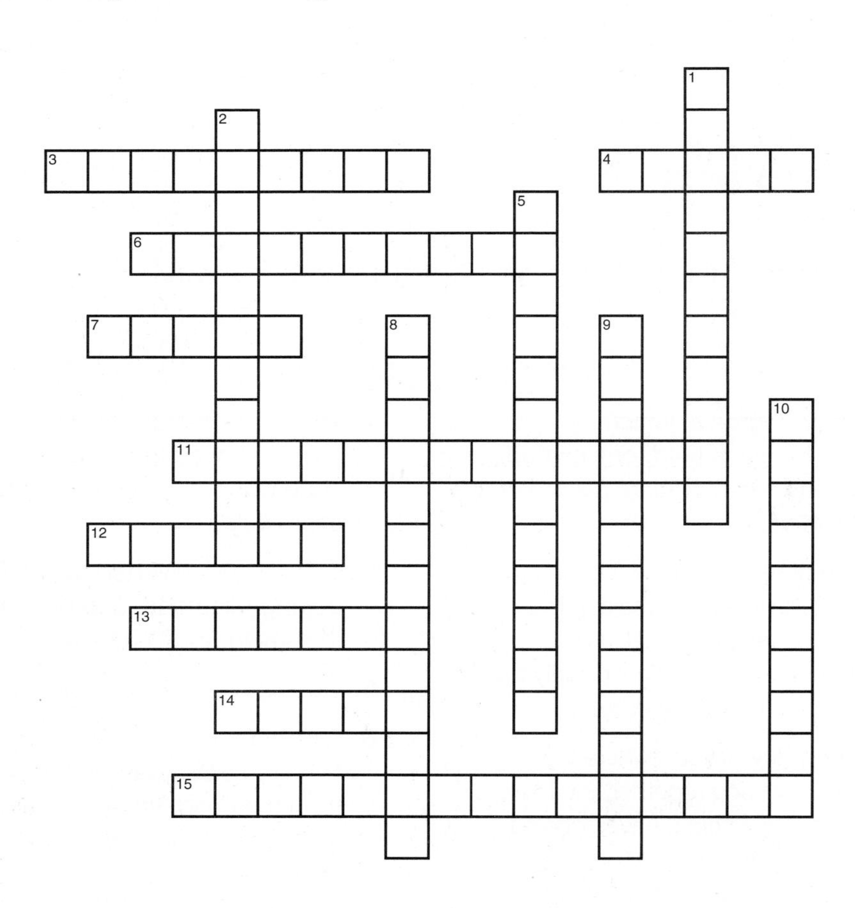

CHAPTER 15 MEN'S HAIR REPLACEMENT

LEARNING OBJECTIVES

After completing this chapter, you will be able to:

LO1 Discuss the reasons why men may purchase a hair replacement system.

LO2 Understand the factors that influence hair replacement systems.

LO3 Discuss selling hair replacement systems.

LO4 Discuss alternative hair replacement methods.

LO5 Identify the types of hair used in hair replacement systems.

LO6 Define stock and custom replacement systems.

LO7 Recognize supplies needed to service hair replacement systems.

LO8 Describe how to clean and service a hair replacement system.

LO9 Describe how to fit and cut in a hair replacement system.

Introduction

LO1 Discuss the reasons why men may purchase a hair replacement system.

Short Answer/Fill-in-the-Blank

1 List three reasons why studying men's hair replacement is important for a barber.

a. ______________________________

____

____

b. ______________________________

____

____

c. ______________________________

____

____

2 During the eighteenth century, the word ______________ was used to describe the front section of hair, also known as the ______________.

3 Hair replacement options range from topical applications of drugs such as ______________ to hair replacement systems to surgical hair ______________ and scalp ______________.

Why Study Men's Hair Replacement?

Multiple Choice

4 Barbers should have a thorough understanding of men's hair replacement because:

a. They will have more confidence.

b. It will make clients more talkative.

c. It can lead to increased clientele and financial gain.

d. It is a requirement of state barber boards.

Mastering the Art of the Consultation

LO 2 **Understand the factors that influence hair replacement systems.**

Fill-in-the-Blank

5 When discussing hair replacement with your client, you should be sure to take a very ______________________ and ______________________ approach.

6 Take the time during the consultation to explain the finer points of hair restoration, ______________________, ______________________ methods, and different hair ______________________.

7 You can determine how many ______________________ your client will need by his ______________________, age, as well as the amount of money he is willing to spend.

Selling Hair Replacement Systems

LO 3 **Discuss selling hair replacement systems.**

True or False

8 For the following statements, circle T if true or F if false.

T **F** When a man expresses an interest in wearing a hair solution to his barber, he will appreciate a hard-sell approach.

T **F** The barber should never raise the client's expectations to an unreasonable level.

T **F** Dark, opaque colors are recommended for any age group, especially older persons.

T **F** The more natural looking the color, the less obvious the hair solution will appear.

Marketing and Display Techniques

Short Answer

9 Write a tip or guideline for each of the marketing and display techniques below.

a. Social Media Marketing Techniques

b. Hair Replacement System Display

c. Referrals and Word of Mouth

d. Window Displays

e. Personal Approach

f. Print Ads

____

____

____

____

____

g. Personal Experience

____

____

____

____

____

Understand Alternative Hair Replacement Methods

LO 4 **Discuss alternative hair replacement methods.**

Nonsurgical and Surgical Options

Matching

10 Match the correct hair replacement method with each description.

_____ Removal of the bald scalp area and attachment of hair-bearing skin

_____ Side effects can include weight gain and loss of sexual function

_____ Can be offered in the barbershop

_____ Removal of hair from normal-growth areas of the scalp and transplantation into the bald areas

_____ Oral medication that is prescribed only for men

_____ Use of a cold-beam, red-light laser to stimulate or increase blood circulation

_____ Removal of bald area from the scalp, withhair growth pulled together to fill in the spot

_____ Available for both men and women in a 2 percent formula

a. Finasteride

b. Flap surgery

c. Laser therapy

d. Minoxidil

e. Hair transplantation

f. Scalp reduction

Learn about Hair Replacement Systems

LO 5 Identify the types of hair used in hair replacement systems.

LO 6 Define stock and custom replacement systems.

Human, Synthetic, and Mixed Hair

Case Study/Fill-in-the-Blank

11 Hair Used for Hair Replacement

Clients may be interested in purchasing a hair replacement system but may not be aware of their options or what option to choose. Therefore, it is important for a barber who specializes in hair replacement systems to inform clients of the best solution for them. Imagine a client decides to purchase a hair replacement system. Explain the advantages and disadvantages of hair replacement systems made of human hair, synthetic hair, and mixed hair.

____

____

____

____

____

____

____

____

____

____

____

____

____

____

____

12 ____________________ hair has become the most popular choice when it comes to hair replacement.

13 ____________________ is the process used to comb through the hair strands of a hair solution to separate them.

Understand Bases and Construction

Fill-in-the-Blank

14 Hair replacement systems are available with ______________________, ______________________, ______________________, ______________________, ______________________, or ______________________ bases.

15 Some professionals prefer a ______________________ base material for increased strength and ______________________.

16 ______________________ refers to the way the hair is attached to the base of the hair solution.

17 ______________________ refers to sorting the hair strands so that the cuticle points toward the hair ends in its natural direction of growth, thus minimizing ______________________ and ______________________.

Understand Stock and Custom Hair Replacement Systems

Fill-in-the-Blank

18 ______________________ can be used as samples to show prospective hair replacement clients what a replacement system might look like or may be customized to fit the client if one happens to be the correct color.

19 A ______________________ or ______________________ analysis should be done prior to fitting any hair solution.

Obtaining Hair Replacement Systems

LO 7 **Recognize supplies needed to service hair replacement systems.**

Short Answer

20 What are four sample questions that help when selecting a manufacturer to provide hair replacement goods for a barbershop?

- ____
- ____
- ____
- ____

Supplies for Hair Replacement Services

Word Search

21 Find the ten hair solution service supplies and circle them in the word search below.

T	O	E	T	V	S	E	R	I	V
P	C	N	A	L	C	O	H	O	L
I	I	V	L	O	N	O	C	E	I
N	P	E	P	S	R	A	Z	O	R
S	C	L	I	P	P	E	R	S	O
B	L	O	W	D	R	Y	E	R	C
R	S	P	I	R	I	T	G	U	M
D	E	E	S	O	L	V	E	N	T
I	A	S	C	I	S	S	O	R	S
A	D	H	E	S	I	V	E	D	V

1. adhesive
2. alcohol
3. blowdryer
4. clippers
5. envelopes
6. razor
7. scissors
8. solvent
9. spirit gum
10. T-pins

Measure and Mold for Hair Replacement Systems

Fill-in-the-Blank

22 When performing the ________________________ cut, the hair should be lightly trimmed, leaving a long ________________________ and length close to the ________________________ at the sides.

23 Take a separate ________________________ from the temple, side, and back area if the client has ________________________ hair to ensure the correct blend of color at the blending area of the system.

24 Custom pieces require a ________________________ or ________________________ of the client's head form in the area of hair loss.

25 Some manufacturer's prefer ________________________ models of the client's head form.

Discuss Ways to Affix Hair Replacement Systems

Matching

26 Match the correct hair replacement attachment process with each description.

_____ Attached with spirit gum

_____ Can be made for the front or crown areas of the head

_____ Held in place by permanent elastic bands at the sides

_____ Uses an adhesive bonding agent to adhere to all areas of the head, rather than tape alone

_____ Recommended when the hair is worn in an off-the-face style

a. Full head bonding
b. Partial hair replacement systems
c. Lace-front hair solution
d. Facial hair replacement solutions
e. Full wigs

Cleaning and Styling Hair Replacement Systems

LO 8 **Describe how to clean and service a hair replacement system.**

LO 9 **Describe how to fit and cut in a hair replacement system.**

Cleaning Synthetic Hair Replacement Systems

Fill-in-the-Blanks

27 Synthetic hair solutions should always be cleaned with ______________.

28 Do not use ______________, which could cause the hair solution to ______________ or become matted and tangled.

29 Fill in the blanks to complete the procedure for cleaning human hair replacement systems.

1. Remove all the ______________ and clean any reinforced areas by lightly dabbing with the recommended ______________.
2. Put enough ______________ in a glass bowl so that the hair system can be ______________. Invert the hair replacement with the inside up and place into the cleaning solution. Soak for ______________ minutes.
3. Gently ______________ the edge of the hair replacement with a small ______________ or your fingers until the ______________ has been removed.
4. Place a ______________ on a flat surface and place the hair replacement on the towel with the ______________ facing up. Gently press out the ______________ with the towel.
5. Hold the replacement by the ______________ section and ______________ gently.
6. Fasten the replacement to the ______________ with T-pins, style with a ______________, and store until the client picks it up, or dry the hair replacement and reattach to client's ______________.

30 Fill in the blanks to complete the procedure for cleaning wigs.

1. ______________ the wig thoroughly to remove all ______________ dirt and residue.
2. Mix a solution of ______________ water and wig ______________ in a bowl.
3. ______________ the entire wig into the solution; swish it around in the solution.
4. Rinse the wig in clean, ______________ water.
5. Blot it dry with a ______________.
6. Turn the wig ______________ and dry it with a towel.
7. Pin the wig to a ______________ or ______________ of the correct size.
8. Carefully ______________ the hair into place.
9. Permit the wig to dry ______________, pinned to the form.
10. If necessary, use ______________ air to dry the wig quickly.
11. When ______________, brush into the proper style.

Basic Hair Replacement System Care

Short Answer

31 List four guidelines for basic hair replacement system care.

- ____
  ____
  ____
- ____
  ____
  ____
- ____
  ____
  ____
- ____
  ____
  ____

Recondition and Permanent Waving Hair Replacement Systems

Fill-in-the-Blank

32 Reconditioning treatments should be given as often as necessary to prevent ______________ or ______________ of the hair.

33 If a slight color adjustment is necessary due to fading or ______________, a suitable ______________ is recommended.

34 The objective when permanent waving a hair solution is to create ______________ that blends the system with the client's natural hair.

35 The rod placement does not rest on the scalp of the hair system; instead, the rods are ______________ to eliminate weight and ______________ on the base.

36 Use a ______________ comb with hair replacement systems to avoid weakening or damaging the ______________.

37 Brush and comb hair solutions with a ______________ movement.

Understand Cutting, Tapering, and Blending Hair Replacement Systems

Multiple Choice

38 When removing bulk from a hair solution, make ______________ partings in order to keep it looking natural.

a. the fewest

b. very narrow

c. very wide

d. very precise

39 After cutting and blending a full head bonded replacement system, remember to tell the client to allow ______________ before shampooing.

a. 24 to 48 hours

b. 12 hours

c. 30 minutes

d. 3 to 4 days

Word Review

Matching

Draw a line connecting each term with its definition.

Finasteride	The process of attaching a hair replacement system to all areas of the head with an adhesive bonding agent.
Flap surgery	The surgical removal of a bald area, followed by the pulling together of the scalp ends.
Full head bonding	Any form of hair restoration that involves the surgical removal and relocation of hair, including scalp reduction and flap surgery.
Hackling	Also known as *styling block*; a head-shaped form made of plastic, foam, or other materials used as a stand for a wig or hair replacement system.
Hair replacement system	A process used to comb through the hair strands to separate them.
Hair solution	An oral medication prescribed for men only to stimulate hair growth.
Hair transplantation	Refers to sorting the hair strands so that the cuticle points toward the hair ends in its natural direction of growth.
Lace-front	A surgical technique that involves the removal of a bald scalp area and the attachment of a flap of hair-bearing skin.
Minoxidil	A popular hair solution style used for off-the-face styles.
Root-turning	Formerly called a *hairpiece*; also known as a hair solution.
Scalp reduction	A topical medication used to promote hair growth or reduce hair loss.
Toupee	Any small wig used to cover the top or crown of the head and integrated with the natural hair.
Wig block	An outdated term used to describe a small hair replacement that covers the top or crown of the head.

CHAPTER 16 WOMEN'S HAIRCUTTING AND STYLING

LEARNING OBJECTIVES

After completing this chapter, you will be able to:

LO1 **Identify the differences between men's and women's haircutting.**

LO2 **Describe four basic women's haircuts.**

LO3 **Explain wave formation in curly hair textures.**

LO4 **Discuss other haircutting techniques.**

LO5 **Explain different hairstyling techniques.**

LO6 **Demonstrate a blunt cut.**

LO7 **Demonstrate a graduated cut.**

LO8 **Demonstrate a uniform-layered cut.**

LO9 **Demonstrate a long-layered cut.**

Introduction

Short Answer/Fill-in-the-Blank

1 List three reasons why studying women's haircutting and styling is important for a barber.

a. ____

____

____

b. ____

____

____

c. ____

____

____

2 If you choose to work in a ____________________, it is a must to be proficient in cutting and styling women's hair.

3 Styling women's hair tends to be a more involved process than styling men's hair and includes techniques such as ____________________, ____________________, and styling with a ____________________ or ____________________.

Why Study Women's Haircutting and Styling?

Multiple Choice

4 Barbers should have a thorough understanding of women's haircutting and styling because:

a. A woman may request a service.

b. It is required to obtain a barbering license.

c. More women are now frequenting barbershops than men.

d. It is easier to cut and style women's hair than men's.

Discuss Men's versus Women's Haircutting

LO 1 **Identify the differences between men's and women's haircutting.**

Multiple Choice

5 Shorter, tapered men's cuts usually appear ________________ on a woman.

a. longer

b. shorter

c. straighter

d. more angular

6 In women's haircutting, curved design lines, feathering, or texturizing at the perimeter is often used to ________________ the look of a short cut.

a. harden

b. soften

c. angle

d. square up

7 Women's cuts tend to require more ________________ than men's cuts to achieve the final look.

a. styling

b. hot towels

c. mirrors

d. razor work

Haircutting Reminders

Fill-in-the-Blank/Short Answer

8 Complete the following rules for cutting women's hair.

- Start with clean, ________________ hair.
- Take consistent, clean ________________ to produce precise results.
- Keep the hair ________________ when cutting.
- Work with the natural ________________, not against them.
- Use the appropriate amount of ________________ when combing and holding sections of hair, as determined by the hair ________________.
- Always work with a ________________ or ________________.
- Plan for the ________________ factor that results when the hair dries or when cutting ________________ and ________________ hair textures.
- Always check and ________________ your work.

9 Cross-checking is the process of checking your work. Explain briefly how to cross-check.

Define Four Basic Women's Haircuts

LO 2 Describe four basic women's haircuts.

Blunt, Graduated, Uniform-Layered, and Graduated Haircuts

Fill-in-the-Blank/Matching

10 Identify the haircuts in the images below.

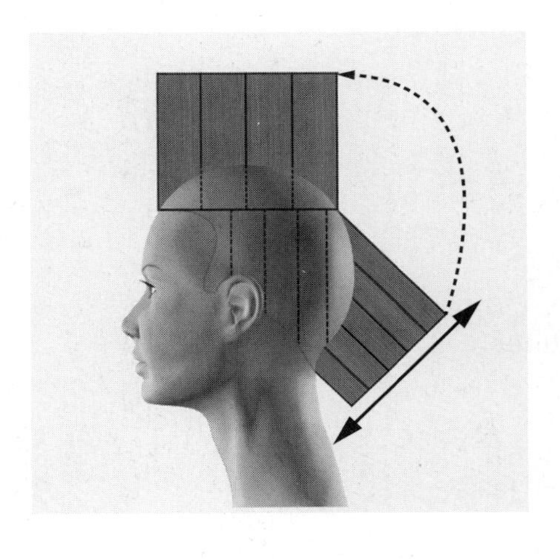

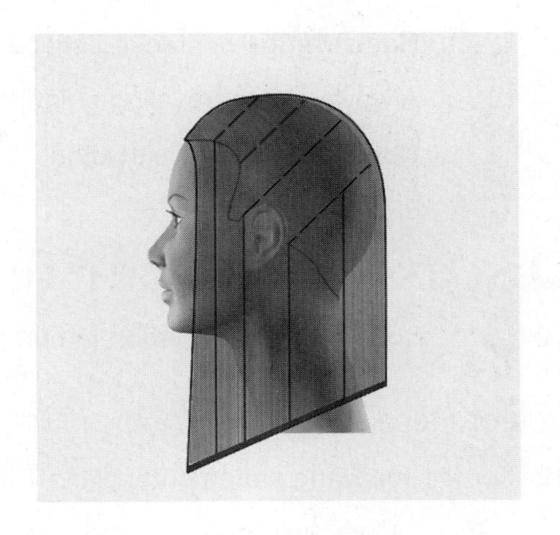

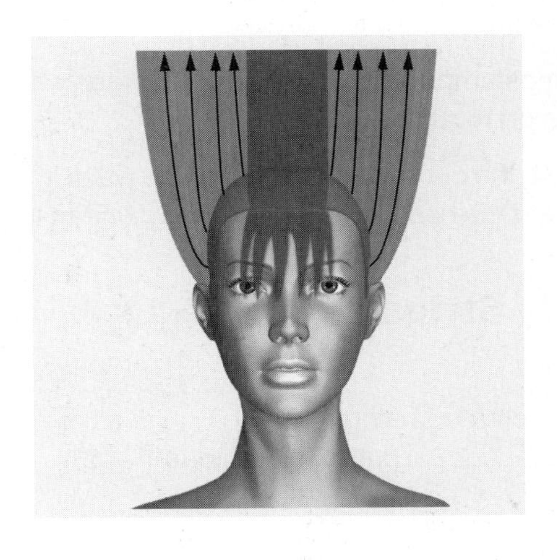

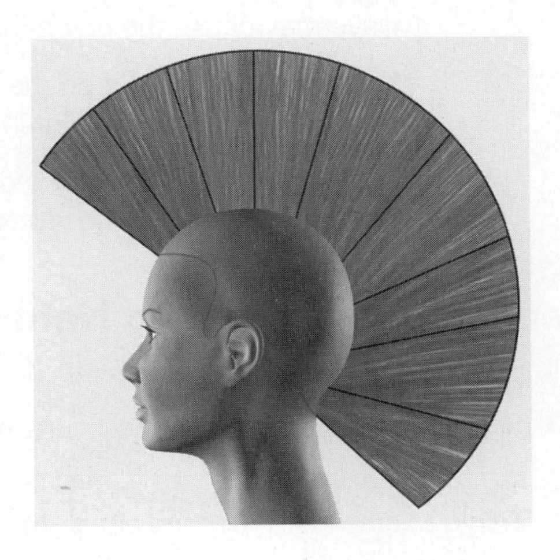

11 Match the correct haircut with each description.

_____	Finished look is soft and textured and conforms to the head shape without lines or corners	**a. Blunt**
_____	Cut at 45-degree elevation	**b. Graduated**
_____	Also known as a *one-length*	**c. Long-layered**
_____	Produces progressively longer layers from the top to the perimeter	**d. Uniform-layered**
_____	Cut at 0-degree elevation	
_____	Sometimes begins with a stationary guide in the top section of the head	
_____	Builds weight and volume along the perimeter	
_____	Cut at 90-degree elevation	
_____	Head should be held upright to avoid shifting the hair out of natural fall	
_____	Has a wedge or stacked shape	
_____	Always uses a traveling guide	
_____	Cut at 180-degree elevation	

Discuss Curly Hair Textures

LO 3 **Explain wave formation in curly hair textures.**

True or False

12 For the following statements, circle T if true or F if false.

T **F** Curly hair tends to graduate naturally due to the elasticity and curl pattern.

T **F** Depending on the amount of curl, cutting the hair parting in the trough of the wave may cause the hair ends to fall inward toward the head form.

T **F** Knowing where to cut on the wave is most important when cutting longer hairstyles, especially maintenance cuts on regular customers.

T **F** Cutting a little less or a little more will place the cut line at the crest of the wave again and encourage the hair to curl toward the head form instead of away from it.

Techniques for Cutting Natural Curly Styles

Fill-in-the-Blank

13 Short natural cuts on extremely curly hair can be created using the _______________ or _______________ cutting technique.

14 Thick, coarse hair types are easier to cut with _______________.

15 Curly hair of _______________ density and a _______________ curl may be easier to cut with shears.

16 The curlier the hair, the more it will ______________________ as it dries and give the appearance of a change in ____________________.

Explore Various Cutting Techniques

LO 4 Discuss other haircutting techniques.

Overdirection, Razor Cutting, and Texturizing

Matching

17 Match the description with the correct haircutting technique.

_____ Used to increase the lengths in a perimeter design line	**a. Overdirection**
_____ Uses a sliding shears movement to thin the hair to graduated lengths	**b. Razor cutting**
_____ Creates separation in the hair	**c. Point cutting**
_____ Creates a chunky effect	**d. Notching**
_____ Produces an angle at the ends of the hair	**e. Slithering**
_____ Performed at the ends of the hair using the tips of the shears at a steep shear angle	**f. Slicing**
_____ Blades are kept open, and only the portion of the blade near the pivot is used for cutting	**g. Carving**

Discuss Hairstyling

LO 5 Explain different hairstyling techniques.

Case Study

18 Styling Women's Hair

The first step in the hairstyling process is the client consultation. During the consultation, the client should be guided toward the most suitable hairstyle for her face shape, hair texture, and lifestyle. What hairstyle would you suggest for a client who has thick, naturally curly (but not very curly) hair and wants a straight, smooth look?

____

____

____

____

____

____

____

____

____

Wet Hairstyling

Crossword Puzzle

19 Fill in the correct term in the crossword puzzle using the clues provided.

Across

Clue

6. Performed with Marcel irons or electric thermal (curling) irons.
8. Technique used to keep curly hair smooth and straight while retaining a beautiful shape.
9. Technique of drying and styling damp or wet hair in one step.
10. Uses heat to produce curls or waves or straightened hair.
11. Temporarily straightens hair by using heated pressing combs or irons.

Down

Clue

1. Set a pattern in the hair that will form the basis for a hairstyle.
2. Process of combing the hair straight down over the client's head, followed by drying, and finishing with thermal irons.
3. Process of shaping and directing the hair into an S-shaped pattern through the use of fingers, comb, and setting lotion.
4. Used to give direction to straighter hair texture styles while imparting a glossy, finished look to the hair.
5. Towel-dried hair is combed into place or arranged into a style with the hands and fingers, then allowed to dry.
7. Wound from the hair ends into a spiral or circle creating a flattened curl formation against the head.

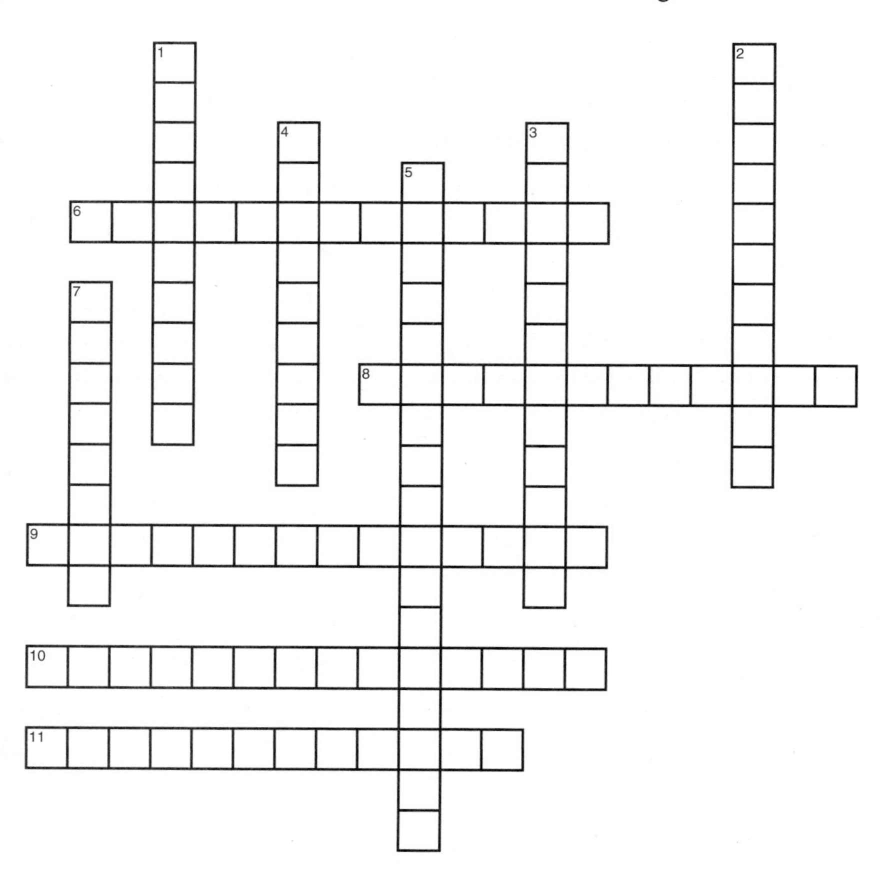

Blunt Cut

LO 6 **Demonstrate a blunt cut.**

Fill-in-the-Blank

20 Fill in the blanks to complete the steps from the blunt cut procedure.

6. Starting in the center, using the ____________ teeth, comb the hair into ____________ and cut line parallel to the ____________ forward parting. Repeat on the opposite side, starting cut from the outer corner to the center creating a slight arc-shaped line.

7. Take another set of ____________ forward partings from the top of the occipital to the top of each ear. Take a ____________ part that runs from the front hairline to the nape, dividing the head into two. The head ____________ will move up slightly, but the natural fall distribution and ____________-degree elevation remain consistent. Cut parallel to parting and follow the length of your guide.

8. With the client's head ____________, take a ____________ section from just below the crown to the front hairline. Starting in the rear of the ____________ section, using the ____________ teeth, comb the hair into ____________ over the previously cut hair. Cut the line along the comb following your guide beneath, till you reach the sides just below the ear.

9. On the sides just behind the ear, continue to comb the hair to ____________, cutting the hair ____________ to the horseshoe parting.

10. Repeat on the opposite side.

11. Take another subsection from the ____________ above the crown to the front hairline. Starting at the ____________, comb the hair to ____________ and cut at ____________ elevation following your guide. When you reach the sides continue the same technique as Step 9.

12. Release the remainder of the section, comb hair to ____________, paying close attention to any cowlicks or movement at the crown. Starting at the ____________ continue combing the hair to ____________ and cutting at ____________ elevation following your guide.

13. To check the line for accuracy, ____________ hair straight and smooth sectioning the hair the same way it was cut, using ____________ brush.

Graduated Cut

LO 7 **Demonstrate a graduated cut.**

Fill-in-the-Blank

21 Fill in the blanks to complete the steps from the graduated cut procedure.

18. In preparation for ____________, create a radial section by taking a ____________ parting from the ____________ to the top of each ear. Take a ____________-wide central vertical subsection from the crown to the ____________.

19. The hair in this section is elevated to ________________ degrees and ________________ back. Your guide will be taken from the ________________ of the graduation for the length. You will ________________ following the head shape.

20. ________________ subsections are combed to ________________ degrees, ________________ back, and, using a traveling guide, cut parallel to the head. When you have completed the radial section, repeat on the opposite side.

21. When you reach the sides, take a ________________ subsection from the natural ________________ part, elevate to ________________ degrees, overdirect back, and ________________ following your guide from the ________________ section.

22. In the front, ________________ is maintained by overdirecting back to a ________________ guide at the radial section. Repeat the same steps on the opposite side.

23. Once the hair is dry, detail the ________________, starting at the ________________, use the points of your shears for softness or blunt cut for a stronger line. At the sides, clean up your line at the perimeter.

Uniform-Layered Cut

LO 8 **Demonstrate a uniform-layered cut.**

Fill-in-the-Blank

22 Fill in the blanks to complete the steps from the uniform-layered cut procedure.

6. Starting at the ________________, elevate the hair to ________________ degrees and cut ________________ inches in length working in small increments following the head shape.

7. Above ________________, switch hand position and cut to the ________________ knuckle to avoid ________________ forming on the line. Follow the guide to the front hairline. Once you have cut the center guide, check the length for balance and remove any corners.

8. After completing the guide, make a ________________ section from recession to recession and below the ________________. Make sure your section is clean and ________________ at both sides of the recession.

9. Take a ________________ parting from the occipital to the back of each ear and ________________ the section above your ________________ line. At the back, take a center section from the ________________ to the nape dividing your first initial profile section ________________ into half.

10. Starting at the ________________ back, take a slight ________________ forward parting through to the nape, ________________ your guide from the profile section.

11. Elevate the hair to ________________ degrees and cut parallel to the parting for your subsection following the guide. (________________ position is ________________ when cutting the left side.)

12. ________________ horizontally; on every ________________ section, the line should go ________________ because you are following the head shape.

Long-Layered Cut

LO 9 **Demonstrate a long-layered cut.**

Multiple Choice

23 After taking a central profile parting from the front hairline through to the nape, take two slight diagonal forward subsections (________________ wide) from the occipital to behind the ear.

a. ½ inch
b. 1 inch
c. 2 inches
d. 3 inches

24 For the perimeter guide, starting in the center back, comb the hair to natural fall at ________________ degrees and cut (length) the line parallel to the parting.

a. 0
b. 45
c. 90
d. 180

25 On the sides, comb the hair to natural fall and ________________ to behind the shoulder and cut the line square to your guide.

a. point cut
b. underdirect
c. slither
d. overdirect

26 To keep the length on the sides from front to back, avoid cutting the corner at the sideburn area or just ________________.

a. next to the eyes
b. at the shoulder
c. in front of the ear
d. behind the ear

27 Starting at the front hairline, take a ________________ profile section to the occipital, using your length from the chin as a guide.

a. ½ inch
b. 1-inch
c. 2-inch
d. 3-inch

Word Review

Short Answer

Fill in the definition for the following terms.

Blunt cut

Circle

Graduated cut

Hair pressing

Long-layered cut

Off-base

Stem

Thermal styling

Uniform-layered cut

CHAPTER 17 CHEMICAL TEXTURE SERVICES

LEARNING OBJECTIVES

After completing this chapter, you will be able to:

LO1 Describe how permanent waves, relaxers, and curl reformation services change the appearance of the hair.

LO2 List topics to discuss during a client consultation.

LO3 Identify six characteristics of the hair and scalp that are analyzed before performing chemical texturizing services.

LO4 Describe how the ingredients in permanent waves, relaxers, and curl reformation services are chemically similar and chemically different from each other.

LO5 Explain the physical and chemical actions of permanent waving, chemical relaxing, and curl reformation processes.

LO6 Identify types of perm rods and end wrapping techniques.

LO7 Define *on-base, half off-base,* and *off-base* rod placement.

LO8 Identify two types of chemical relaxers.

LO9 Explain the difference between *base* and *no-base* relaxers.

LO10 List three strand tests to be performed before a chemical relaxing process.

LO11 Explain the three steps of a curl reformation process.

LO12 Describe the intended outcomes of texturizer and chemical blowout services.

Introduction

Short Answer/Fill-in-the-Blank

1 List the reasons studying chemical texture services is important for a barber.

a. ______________________________

____

____

b. ______________________________

____

____

c. ______________________________

____

____

d. ______________________________

____

____

2 Chemical texture services, such as permanent waving (also known as chemical waving), curl reformations, and relaxers, chemically change the hair's natural ______________________.

3 Clients with naturally overly curly hair may straighten their hair by having it chemically ______________________.

Why Study Chemical Texture Services?

Multiple Choice

4 Barbers should have a thorough understanding of chemical texture services because:

- **a.** It will result in paying less taxes.
- **b.** Booth rent will be lower.
- **c.** Clients will request services that require no maintenance.
- **d.** Barbers may be expected to provide these services.

Learn about Chemical Texture Services

LO 1 **Describe how permanent waves, relaxers, and curl reformation services change the appearance of the hair.**

Multiple Choice/Fill-in-the-Blank/Case Study

5 The processes for a ______________________ require a thio-based waving lotion.

- **a.** permanent wave and relaxer
- **b.** chemical relaxer and curl reformation
- **c.** curl reformation and permanent wave
- **d.** curl rejuvenation and reformation

6 The process for a ______________________ may include a sodium hydroxide relaxer.

- **a.** permanent wave
- **b.** chemical relaxer
- **c.** curl reformation
- **d.** curl rejuvenation

7 A curl reformation is a combination of a thio-based chemical ______________________ and a permanent ______________________ .

8 ______________________ is a process used to chemically restructure natural hair into a different wave pattern.

9 **Chemical Texture Service Comparison**

Some clients want their hair to look different, such as curlier or straighter, but may not know exactly what texture service to request. Some clients even use the term *perm* when they are referring to a relaxer. Barbers must be able to educate clients about the products and services available for hair and clear up misconceptions and confusion. How would you compare permanent wave, relaxer, and curl reformation services toa client?

____

____

____

____

____

Discuss Client Consultation and Analysis

LO 2 **List topics to discuss during a client consultation.**

LO 3 **Identify six characteristics of the hair and scalp that are analyzed before performing chemical texturizing services.**

Short Answer

10 List five topics to discuss during a client consultation:

1. ______________________________

2. ______________________________

3. ______________________________

4. ______________________________

5. ______________________________

Understand Scalp and Hair Analysis

Short Answer/Matching/True or False

11 List six characteristics of the hair that are determined prior to performing chemical texturizing services.

1. ______________________________

2. ______________________________

3. ______________________________

4. ______________________________

5. ______________________________

6. ______________________________

12 Match the following characteristics with the correct term. Terms may be used more than once.

_____ Has a raised cuticle layer

_____ Neither resistant nor overly porous

_____ Tight, compact cuticle layer

_____ Requires a more alkaline solution

_____ Services usually process as expected

_____ Absorbs chemical solutions easily

_____ Inhibits penetration of chemical solutions

_____ Requires a less alkaline solution

a. Resistant

b. Normal

c. Porous

13 Explain how to perform a porosity test.

____

____

____

____

____

____

____

14 For the following statements, circle T if true or F if false.

T **F** Hair texture helps determine the amount of product to use.

T **F** The greater the degree of elasticity, the longer the wave will remain in the hair.

T **F** Hair density helps determine the number of blockings or subsections that will be best for the service that is performed.

T **F** In permanent waving and curl reformation processes, hair length may determine the wrapping technique to use.

15 Explain how to perform an elasticity test.

____

____

____

____

____

Understand the Chemistry of Chemical Texture Services

LO 4 **Describe how the ingredients in chemical waves, relaxers, and curl reformation services are chemically similar and chemically different from each other.**

LO 5 **Explain the physical and chemical actions of permanent waving, chemical relaxing, and curl reformation processes.**

Fill-in-the-Blank

16 Chemical texture services create ____________________ changes in the structure and appearance of the hair.

17 The two layers of the hair most affected by chemical texture services are the ____________________ and ____________________.

18 The degree to which hair is resistant to chemical changes depends on the strength of the ____________________.

19 The ______________________ gives the hair its strength, flexibility, elasticity, and shape.

20 Chemical bonds in the cortex are ______________________ with chemical texture services.

Define the Principle Actions of Chemical Texturizing Services

Fill-in-the-Blank

21 Thio relaxing products also require the use of a ______________________ to chemically oxidize the hair.

22 The neutralizer for permanent waves neutralizes any remaining waving lotion in the hair through ______________________.

23 A ______________________ action of the permanent wave involves wrapping the hair around permrods.

24 The ______________________ for a curl reformation relaxes the natural curl by softening and swelling the cuticle, allowing for penetration into the ______________________.

25 Most thio relaxers have a pH above ______________________ and are manufactured in cream form for better adhesion and control.

26 Hydroxide relaxing products are neutralized through the physical actions of the ______________________ and ______________________ process because the disulfide bonds that have been broken by this type of relaxer cannot be reformed through oxidation.

Know about Permanent Waves

LO 6 **Identify types of perm rods and end wrapping techniques.**

LO 7 **Define *on-base, half off-base,* and *off-base* rod placement.**

Understand the Chemical Perm Wrap

Matching/Fill-in-the-Blank/Short Answer

27 Match the description of rods with the correct rod type. Terms may be used more than once.

_____ A larger diameter at both ends

_____ Uniform diameter along the length of the rod

_____ The most commonly used permrods

_____ A smaller diameter in the center

_____ Ends together to form a circle

_____ Produce tighter curl in the center

_____ Made of stiff wires covered by soft foam

_____ Used for definite wave pattern, close to the head

_____ Used for a body wave

a. Concave

b. Straight

c. Bender

d. Circle (loop)

28 Identify the end wrapping technique in the images below.

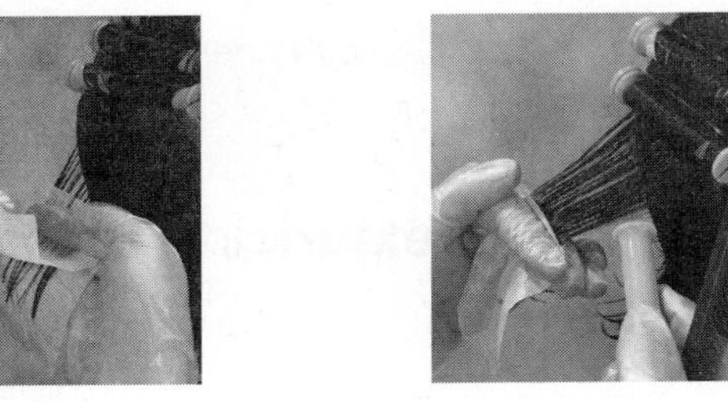

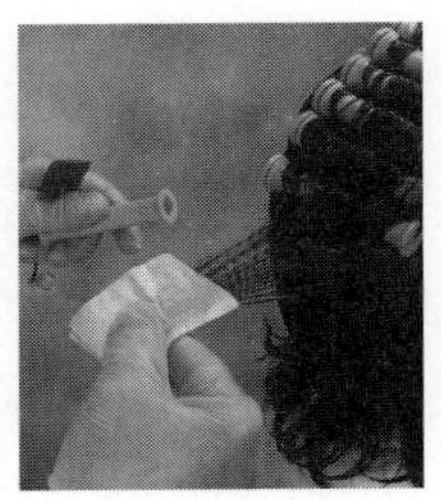

a) ____________________ b) ____________________ c) ____________________

29 Half off-base placement results from wrapping the hair at an angle of ____________________ degrees to its base section.

30 In on-base placement, the hair is projected about ____________________ degrees beyond perpendicular to its base section and the rod is placed ____________________ the base section.

31 Off-base placement is achieved by wrapping the hair at a ____________________degree angle ____________________ perpendicular to its base section.

32 What does *base direction* refer to?

____

____

33 What three partings and positions might be used for rod placement?

____

____

34 In the ____________________ rodding technique, the hair is wound from the ends to the scalp.

35 A ____________________ perm wrap is accomplished by positioning the rod vertically and rodding from the ends to the scalp, or from the scalp to the ends.

36 The two types of wrapping methods used in permanent waving are the ____________________ wrap and the ____________________ wrap.

37 What is the difference between a water wrap and a lotion wrap?

____

____

38 What is the purpose of a lotion wrap? With what type of waving lotion is it used?

____

____

39 The four common wrapping patterns used in permanent waving are the ____________________, ____________________, ____________________, and ____________________ wraps.

Types of Permanent Waves

Short Answer/Fill-in-the-Blank

40 Review the following characteristics of permanent waves, then match to the correct type. Choices may be used more than once.

_____ Main active ingredient is ATG
_____ Most require heat from a blowdryer
_____ Contain sulfates, sulfites, or bisulfites
_____ Used on resistant hair types
_____ Usual pH range of 4.5 to 7.0
_____ Contains an activator with GMTG
_____ Usually marketed as body waves
_____ Strong curl patterns; faster processing time
_____ Produces a softer, natural looking curl
_____ Maintains a constant pH level
_____ Releases heat when mixed
_____ Used on delicate hair types
_____ Usual range of 9.0 to 9.6
_____ Contains ATG and GMTG
_____ Evaporates slowly
_____ May be water or lotion wrapped
_____ Primary reducing agent is GMTG
_____ Produces firmer curls than true-acid waves
_____ Do not produce a firm curl
_____ Has an activator with hydrogen peroxide
_____ Considered to be endothermic perms
_____ Uses alkanolamines
_____ Primary reducing agent is cysteamine or mercaptamine

a. True acid perms
b. Alkaline perms
c. Exothermic waves
d. Acid-balanced waves
e. Thio-free waves
f. Low-pH waves
g. Ammonia-free waves

41 Name three strengths of permanent waving products manufacturers usually produce and the types of hair they are intended for.

a. ____

b. ____

c. ____

42 Resistant hair types usually require an ____________________ wave.

43 ____________________ or ____________________ perms are the usual choice for tinted, highlighted, or delicate hair types.

44 What is a pre-wrap and what does it do?

____

____

Permanent Wave Processing and Wave Formation

Fill-in-the-Blank/Short Answer

45 The amount of processing time depends on the ______________________________ and the ____________________.

46 Most processing takes place within the first ____________________ to ____________________ minutes.

47 The wave has reached its peak when it forms a firm letter ____________________ shape.

48 Frizziness when dry is an indication of ____________________.

49 A weak wave formation is an indication of ____________________.

50 What is the purpose of a test curl? ______________________________

____

51 What important aspects of a permanent wave service can be observed from a test curl?

- ______________________________
- ______________________________
- ______________________________
- ______________________________
- ______________________________

Neutralization

Short Answer/Fill-in-the-Blank

52 What are neutralizers?

____

____

53 The most common neutralizer is ____________________.

54 What are two important functions of a neutralizer?

____

____

55 What important step should be included in the neutralization process after the waving lotion has been rinsed from the hair? Why?

____

____

56 A mild ____________________ shampoo and a ____________________ conditioner should be recommended for permed hair.

Partial Perms, Special Problems, and Safety Precautions

Fill-in-the-Blank

57 When only a portion of the hair is permed, it is called a ____________________.

58 ____________________ treatments should be given to dry, damaged hair prior to a permanent wave service.

59 Fill in the blanks to complete the following safety precautions associated with permanent waving.

- **a.** Always protect clients clothing with a ____________________ drape.
- **b.** Use two towels; one ____________________ the cape and one over the cape.
- **c.** Always examine the client's ____________________ before a perm service.
- **d.** Do not perm excessively ____________________ hair or hair that has been treated with ____________________ relaxers.
- **e.** Always apply a ____________________ barrier around the client's hairline before applying the waving solution.
- **f.** Immediately replace ____________________ cotton coils or towels.
- **g.** Always protect the client's ____________________ with a towel when applying waving and neutralizing solutions.
- **h.** Do not ____________________ or ____________________ to solutions unless specified by the manufacturer.
- **i.** Wear ____________________ when applying solutions.
- **j.** Start applications at the crown or top and progress systematically ____________________ each section.
- **k.** Follow the same ____________________ for the neutralizer as used with the waving solution.
- **l.** If it becomes necessary to resaturate the rods during processing, watch the ____________________ development closely.

Know about Chemical Hair Relaxers

LO 8 **Identify two types of chemical relaxers.**

LO 9 **Explain the difference between *base* and *no-base* relaxers.**

LO 10 **List three strand tests to be performed before a chemical relaxing process.**

Types of Relaxers

True or False/Fill-in-the-Blank

60 For the following statements, circle T if true or F if false.

T **F** Hydroxide relaxers are ionic compounds formed by a metal combined with oxygen and hydrogen.

T **F** Neutralizing shampoos or normalizing lotions are basically acid-balanced shampoos that neutralize any remaining sulfide.

T **F** Thio relaxers require the application of a chemical neutralizing solution.

T **F** Thio relaxers usually have a pH above 6.0.

Relaxers

61 ______________________ relaxers contain a base cream that is designed to melt at body temperature and do not require the application of a separate protective base.

62 ______________________ relaxers require the application of a base cream to the entire scalp prior to relaxer application.

Strand Tests for Chemical Relaxers

Short Answer/Fill-in-the-Blank

63 Identify and describe the three types of strand tests.

- ____
- ____
- ____

64 Fill in the blank to describe the procedure for a strand test.

1. Thread a small section of hair through a hole cut into a piece of wax paper or paper towel; do not use ______________________. Do not use a base or cream. Apply ______________________ to the hair section and smooth. Process according to the manufacturer's directions.
2. Thoroughly mist the hair section with ______________________ to remove product and blot.
3. ______________________ with neutralizer or neutralizing shampoo depending on the type of relaxing product used. Check results and make notes on the client record card.
4. If the hair has been satisfactorily straightened, apply ______________________ or ______________________ to the strand, isolate it, and proceed with the relaxing treatment over the remainder of the hair.

Know about Chemical Curl Reformations

LO 11 **Explain the three steps of a curl reformation process.**

True or False/Multiple Choice

65 For the following statements, circle T if true or F if false.

T **F** The last step in the curl reformation process is to wrap the hair on permrods using a thio-based curl booster, much like a permanent wave wrapping procedure.

T **F** The first step in the curl reformation process is to relax the hair into a straighter form using a thio-based rearranger.

T **F** Neutralizing the hair is the second step in the curl reformation process.

66 Which of the following is *not* a product recommended for a curl reformation?

a. Booster.

b. Neutralizer.

c. Rearranger.

d. Powder.

67 The ________________ rebuilds the broken disulfide bonds.

a. booster
b. neutralizer
c. rearranger
d. powder

Understand Texturizers and Chemical Blowouts

LO 12 **Describe the intended outcomes of texturizer and chemical blowout services.**

Fill-in-the-Blank

68 Depending on the ________________ of the thio relaxer, it may not ________________ tightly curled hair textures completely.

69 The primary consideration is to not ________________ the hair to the point where the ________________ process becomes impossible to perform.

70 Check the curl ________________ every few minutes until the desired amount of curl ________________ has been achieved.

Word Review

Matching

_____ A permanent waving wrapping technique in which the waving solution is applied to the section before rodding to pre-soften resistant hair.

_____ Perms that process at room temperature with a pH range of 7.8 to 8.2 do not require hair-dryer heat.

_____ Usually a type of leave-in conditioner applied to the hair prior to permanent waving to equalize porosity.

_____ The position of the wave (perm) rod in relation to its base section.

_____ A process used to semi-straighten extremely curly hair into a more manageable texture and wave pattern.

_____ A combination of a relaxer and hairstyling used to create a variety of Afro styles.

_____ A relaxer with a very high pH, sometimes as high as 13.5.

_____ The process of stopping the action of a permanent wave solution and hardening the hair in its new form by the application of a chemical solution called the neutralizer.

_____ End paper; absorbent papers used to protect and control the ends of the hair during perming services.

a. Acid-balanced waves
b. Base control
c. Chemical blowout
d. End wraps
e. Hydroxide relaxer
f. Lotion wrap
g. Neutralization
h. Pre-wrap solution
i. Texturize

CHAPTER 18

HAIRCOLORING AND LIGHTENING

LEARNING OBJECTIVES

After completing this chapter, you will be able to:

LO1 Identify six hair characteristics that are analyzed before performing haircoloring services.

LO2 Explain color theory principles as they apply to haircolor services.

LO3 Identify haircolor products and explain their actions on hair.

LO4 Explain the action of lighteners on hair.

LO5 Explain procedure and application terms.

LO6 Explain how haircolor products are selected and applied to the hair.

LO7 List haircoloring and lightening safety precautions.

Introduction

Short Answer/Fill-in-the-Blank

1 List four reasons studying haircoloring and lightening is important for a barber.

a. ______________________________

____

____

b. ______________________________

____

____

c. ______________________________

____

____

d. ______________________________

____

____

2 Recently, there has been an increasing demand for ______________ and ______________ coloring.

3 Since the first synthetic dyes were developed in 1883, color technology and haircoloring processes have steadily improved in ______________________ and ______________________.

Why Study Haircoloring and Lightening?

Multiple Choice

4 Barbers should have a thorough understanding of haircoloring and lightening because:

a. It is mandated by the National Association of Barber Boards of America.

b. It will help meet the demand for these services.

c. They are lost arts that can be revitalized.

d. You'll need to teach clients how to perform these techniques at home.

Identify the Characteristics and Structure of Hair

LO 1 **Identify six hair characteristics that are analyzed before performing haircoloring services.**

Short Answer/Matching

5 List six characteristics of the hair that are analyzed prior to performing haircoloring services.

1. ____

2. ____

3. ____

4. ____

5. ____

6. ____

6 Match the following characteristics with the correct term.

_____ Produced by eumelanin and pheomelanin

_____ Determines hair's ability to absorb haircolor products

_____ Classified as fine, medium, or coarse

_____ Determines the subsection size to use for services

_____ An indication of the strength of the cortex

_____ Modified with products to create new colors

a. Elasticity

b. Porosity

c. Density

d. Texture

e. Natural hair color

f. Contributing pigment (undertone)

7 Use the terms *porous*, *low porosity*, *average porosity*, or *high porosity* to identify each characteristic with the correct porosity level.

a. ______________________ Color may fade sooner than other porosity levels

b. ______________________ Permits darker saturation of color

c. ______________________ Hair tends to process in an average amount of time

d. ______________________ Hair that is resistant to chemical penetration

e. ______________________ May require a longer processing time

f. ______________________ Hair that may take color quickly

g. ______________________ Hair with a tight cuticle

h. ______________________ Hair with a slightly raised cuticle

i. ______________________ Accepts Haircolor products faster

j. ______________________ Hair that may not hold color

Understand Color Theory

LO 2 **Explain color theory principles as they apply to haircolor services.**

Primary, Secondary, and Tertiary Colors

Short Answer/Multiple Choice

8 Define each of the following:

a. Primary color: ____

____

b. Secondary color: ____

____

c. Tertiary color: ____

____

9 Which of the following is *not* a primary color?

a. Red.
b. Green.
c. Yellow.
d. Blue.

10 Which of the following is *not* a secondary color?

a. Green.
b. Violet.
c. Orange.
d. Red.

11 Which of the following is *not* a tertiary color?

a. Red-violet.
b. Blue-green.
c. Yellow-orange.
d. Red-blue.

Complementary Colors, Hue, Tone and Level

Fill-in-the-Blank

12 Complementary colors are primary and ____________________ colors positioned directly ____________________ each other on the color wheel.

13 ____________________ describes the warmth or coolness of a color.

14 Level is a unit of measurement used to identify the ____________________ or ____________________ of a color.

15 The ____________________ of a haircoloring product is the predominant tone of a color.

16 Use the image below to determine the complementary color for the following:

COLOR WHEEL

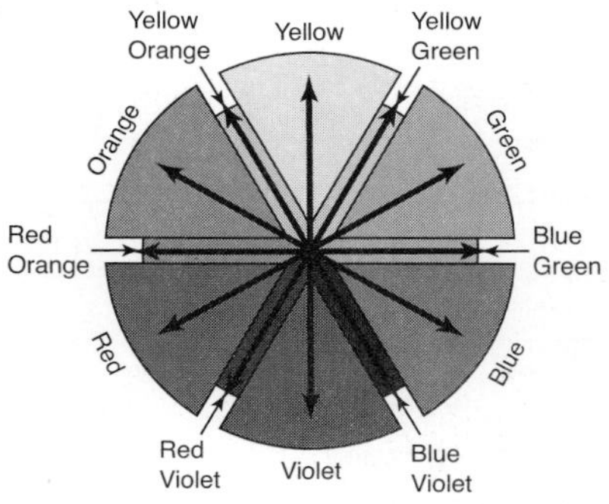

Yellow Orange, Yellow, Yellow Green, Green, Blue Green, Blue, Blue Violet, Violet, Red Violet, Red, Red Orange, Orange

a. Red: ____________________

b. Blue: ____________________

c. Yellow: ____________________

Saturation, Base Color, Natural Level, Tone, and Gray Hair

True or False/Matching/Fill-in-the-Blank

17 For the following statements, circle T if true or F if false.

T **F** The less saturated the product, the more dramatic the change in hair color.

T **F** Artificial haircolors are developed from primary and secondary colors to form "base colors."

T **F** Identifying the natural level and tone of the client's hair will determine which products to use and what the final results will look like.

18 Match the description with the correct base color.

_____	Minimizes orange tones	**a. Violet**
_____	Tends to soften and balance other colors	**b. Blue**
_____	Helps minimize yellow tones	**c. Red-orange**
_____	Creates warm, bright tones in the hair	**d. Neutral**

19 The amount of gray in an individual's hair is measured in ____________________. Identify the percentage of gray indicated by the following conditions.

a. More gray than pigmented: ____________________

b. More pigmented than gray hair: ____________________

c. Virtually no pigmented hair: ____________________

d. Even mixture of gray and pigmented hair: ____________________

Identify Haircoloring Products

LO 3 **Identify haircolor products and explain their actions on hair.**

Fill-in-the-Blank/Short Answer/Multiple Choice

20 Haircoloring products are categorized as ______________________ or ______________________.

21 List four types of haircolor products and explain their differences.

1. ____
____

2. ____
____

3. ____
____

4. ____
____

22 Complete the chart of haircolor-product characteristics. Some answers have been provided to help get you started.

Characteristic	Temporary	Semipermanent	Demipermanent	Permanent
pH	Acid			
Type of reaction (change)		Chemical and physical		
Mixed with hydrogen peroxide (Yes or no?)				Yes
Size/weight of dye molecule			Medium-small	

23 Review the following characteristics of haircoloring products and identify each with the correct type: *Temporary*, *semipermanent*, *demipermanent*, or *permanent* color products.

a. ______________________ Colors with the greatest pigment molecular weight

b. ______________________ Color rinses

c. ______________________ Will last from six to eight shampoos

d. ______________________ Deposits color without lifting

e. ______________________ Usually contains ammonia, oxidative tints, and hydrogen peroxide

f. ______________________ Regarded as the best products for covering gray

g. ______________________ Partially penetrates the hair shaft

h. ______________________ Must be mixed with a low-volume developer

i. ______________________ Can lighten and deposit color in one process

j. ______________________ Coats the outside of the hair strand

k. ______________________ Haircolor sprays

l. ______________________ Considered a penetrating tint

m. ______________________ Chemical composition is acidic

n. ______________________ Typically falls within the 7.0 to 9.0 pH range

o. ______________________ May serve as non-peroxide toner on pre-lightened hair

p. ______________________ Are capable of lifting one or two levels

q. ______________________ Tends to fade with each shampoo

r. ______________________ Referred to as no-lift haircolors

s. ______________________ Requires retouch applications

t. ______________________ Ranges between 9.0 and 10.5 on the pH scale

u. ______________________ Has a pH range of 2.0 to 4.5

v. ______________________ Does not wash out during the shampoo process

w. ______________________ Does not penetrate the cuticle layer

x. ______________________ Color-enhancing shampoo

y. ______________________ Chemical composition is mildly alkaline

z. ______________________ Considered a type of oxidation color

24 An example of a(n) ______________________ is henna.

a. vegetable tint
b. metallic dye
c. oxidation tint
d. compound dye

25 If not used properly, a(n) ______________________ may turn the hair a blackish-gray.

a. vegetable tint
b. metallic dye
c. oxidation tint
d. compound dye

26 When diluted with water and other substances for use in haircoloring, hydrogen peroxide has a mildly acidic pH of ______________________ to ______________________.

27 A hydrogen peroxide volume of ______________________ or more can cause skin irritations, chemical burns, and hair damage.

28 Hydrogen peroxide is distributed for use under a variety of names including ______________________, ______________________, ______________________, and ______________________.

29 Activators are known as ______________________ and ______________________.

30 An activator is an ______________________, consisting of powdered persulfate salts, that is added to haircolors, lighteners, or hydrogen peroxide to increase the ______________________ of the product.

Understand Hair Lighteners

LO 4 **Explain the action of lighteners on hair.**

Multiple Choice/Fill-in-the-Blank/True or False

31 Lighteners change haircolor through a mixture of ______________________.

- **a.** bleach and hydrogen peroxide
- **b.** ammonia and hydrochloric acid
- **c.** bleach and ammonia
- **d.** ammonia and hydrogen peroxide

32 With lighteners, the amount of color change is *not* dependent on which of the following factors?

- **a.** Strength of the lightener.
- **b.** Length of time lightener is on the hair.
- **c.** How much melanin is in the hair.
- **d.** The type of base used.

33 Which of the following *cannot* be accomplished with lighteners?

- **a.** Brighten and lighten an existing shade.
- **b.** Lighten only certain areas of the hair.
- **c.** Remove artificial haircoloring products.
- **d.** Lighten hair without depositing color.

34 ______________________ lighteners contain oxygen-releasing boosters and substances for quick and strong lightening.

- **a.** Oil
- **b.** Powder
- **c.** Cream
- **d.** Gel

35 Use the image below to determine the contributing pigment of the following color levels:

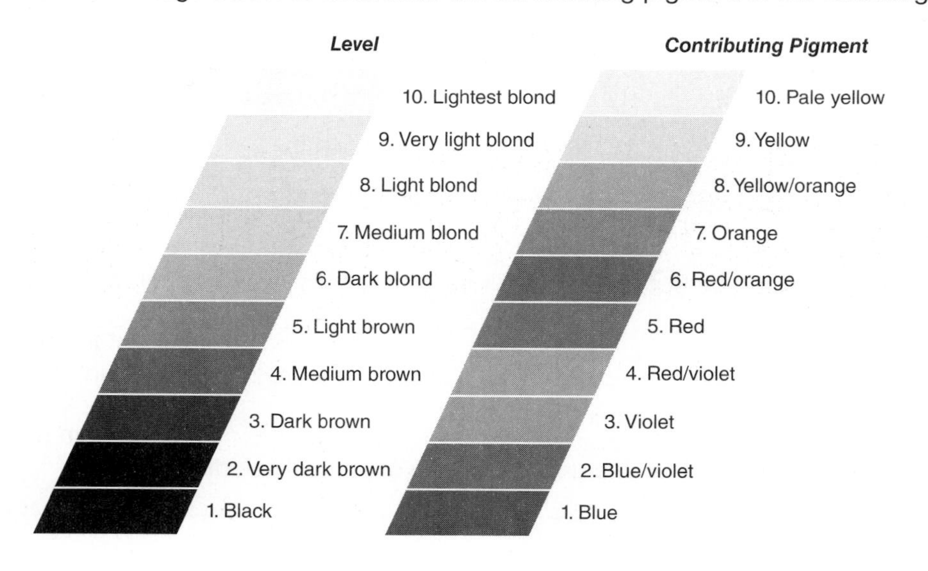

a. Light brown: ______________________

b. Light blond: ______________________

c. Black: ______________________

d. Lightest blond: ______________________

e. Dark brown: ______________________

True or False

36 For the following statements, circle T if true or F if false.

T **F** Toners only add or deposit pigment into the hair shaft; they do not lighten the hair.

T **F** A toner is applied before the lightener application.

T **F** Oil-base dye removers make drastic changes in the level of color.

T **F** Color fillers are dual-purpose haircoloring products that are able to create a color base and equalize excessive porosity in one application.

Understand Procedure and Application Terms

LO 5 **Explain procedure and application terms.**

Short Answer/Fill-in-the-Blank

37 Explain the difference between a virgin application and retouch application.

____

____

38 Explain the procedure for double-process haircoloring.

____

____

39 The ______________________ technique involves pulling strands of hair through the holes of a perforated cap with a hook.

40 The ______________________ technique is the process of painting a lightener or color directly onto clean, styled hair.

41 A soap cap is a combination of equal parts of a permanent haircolor, ______________________, and shampoo that is applied like a regular shampoo.

42 With a tint back, it is important to keep in mind that previously processed hair is more porous and, therefore, may process ______________________ than intended.

43 A client ______________________ should be completed for each client and contain all information pertaining to the haircoloring service.

44 A ______________________ is a form that should be used when the client's hair is in a questionable condition to withstand chemical processes and treatments.

45 Fill in the blanks to complete the steps for performing a haircoloring service client consultation.

1. ____________________ the client.
2. Have the ____________________ fill out the record card.
3. Perform a ____________________ analysis, write the results on a record card, and determine the client's ____________________ color level.
4. Ask ____________________ questions about the desired end result.
5. Show ____________________ of appropriate colors; decide color with the client.
6. Review the procedure, application technique, ____________________, and cost with the client.
7. Perform a ____________________ test if required.
8. Gain approval and begin ____________________.
9. Record end ____________________ on the client record card.

Understand Product Selection and Application

LO 6 **Explain how haircolor products are selected and applied to hair.**

Case Study

46 Selecting Haircolor Products

Imagine you have a middle-aged client who has 50 percent gray hair. Apart from the gray, the hair is one color. The client wants to "get rid" of the gray hair and wants an overall boost in haircolor. The client has never had his hair colored before, and the hair is slightly porous. He is positive of the shade of color he wants. He does not intend to change his mind about the color in the future. Choose the haircolor product(s) that will meet his needs and determine the appropriate level of color increase or reduction.

____

____

____

____

____

Discuss Haircoloring and Lightening Safety Precautions

LO 7 **List haircoloring and lightening safety precautions.**

True or False/Fill-in-the-Blank

47 For the following statements, circle T if true or F if false.

T **F** Off-the-scalp lightener should not be used for virgin or retouch lightener applications.

T **F** Lightener should be applied to the most porous areas first.

T **F** Irritation is a possible result when lightener gets on the towel that is allowed to come in contact with the skin.

48 Work as ________________________ as possible when applying the lightener to produce a ________________________ shade without streaking.

49 Never allow lightener to ________________________; use it immediately.

50 Cap all bottles of developer and lightener to avoid loss of ________________________.

51 Keep a completed ________________________ card of all lightening treatments.

Word Review

Word Search

After identifying the correct terms from the clues provided, locate the terms in the word search.

________________________ A system used to analyze the lightness or darkness of a hair color or color product.

________________________ The predominant tone of an existing color.

________________________ The application of a coloring or lightening product to determine how the hair will react to the formula and the amount of time it will take to process.

________________________ A lightening technique that involves pulling strands of hair through a perforated cap with a plastic or metal hook.

________________________ Deposit-only haircolor product similar to semipermanent but longer lasting.

________________________ A test for identifying a possible allergy to aniline derivative products; required by the FDA 24 to 48 hours before the application of the product.

________________________ The chemical process of diffusing natural or artificial pigment from the hair.

________________________ A term used to describe the warmth or coolness of a color.

______	
______	Powdered persulfate salts added to haircolor to increase its lightening ability.
______	The predominant tone of an existing color.
______	A lightener that cannot be used directly on the scalp.
______	The application of the product to new growth only.
______	Indication that the haircoloring product needs to be applied to the entire hair strand rather than the new growth only.

I	T	T	R	I	T	E	O	N	P	A	T	T	O	L	L	T	I	E	O	N	T
E	I	M	C	L	T	R	I	I	I	P	G	L	T	T	T	O	S	L	F	A	I
T	E	P	S	M	A	E	E	O	U	C	T	E	F	P	C	F	L	A	F	I	P
L	E	R	N	C	O	C	H	O	P	A	O	V	C	R	O	E	C	C	T	O	L
N	A	P	Y	N	N	N	G	A	V	N	A	E	A	C	R	T	E	T	H	O	T
P	H	O	R	F	S	C	E	B	I	S	H	L	P	H	V	M	I	I	E	H	A
H	G	S	C	S	T	R	A	N	D	T	E	S	T	G	I	I	N	V	S	O	C
T	A	I	H	R	O	N	B	R	I	E	G	Y	E	S	R	T	M	A	C	R	B
E	U	I	E	A	N	S	O	C	G	G	A	S	C	A	G	E	C	T	A	T	I
D	E	M	I	P	E	R	M	A	N	E	N	T	H	A	I	R	C	O	L	O	R
G	P	S	H	A	I	R	L	I	G	H	T	E	N	I	N	G	M	R	P	H	D
S	N	T	A	R	H	R	E	B	T	E	E	M	I	C	A	R	C	T	L	H	C
B	T	T	T	I	E	P	O	R	S	C	A	O	Q	S	P	I	A	P	I	E	S
E	A	E	C	Y	R	R	O	M	P	E	Y	B	U	B	P	O	C	A	G	C	E
I	E	S	V	V	V	L	L	O	I	U	I	H	E	N	L	G	E	C	H	N	S
C	H	C	E	L	O	U	E	I	T	O	L	L	M	E	I	N	L	R	T	T	G
O	H	I	R	C	U	H	E	A	T	N	E	O	O	P	C	E	R	C	E	A	L
A	I	R	E	T	O	U	C	H	A	P	P	L	I	C	A	T	I	O	N	A	I
A	A	S	N	A	Y	L	A	I	R	C	L	O	P	A	T	C	H	T	E	S	T
S	A	C	H	H	L	I	O	N	P	T	C	H	S	L	I	A	A	P	R	L	P
B	C	U	A	N	C	M	C	R	C	L	O	N	P	S	O	G	I	Y	T	V	B
U	R	O	L	T	L	P	Q	V	Y	S	N	O	S	V	N	O	N	I	I	G	A

CHAPTER 19

PREPARING FOR LICENSURE AND EMPLOYMENT

LEARNING OBJECTIVES

After completing this chapter, you will be able to:

LO1 Describe the process of taking and passing your state licensing examinations.

LO2 Develop a resume and employment portfolio.

LO3 Know how to explore the job market, research potential employers, and operate within the legal aspects of employment.

Introduction

Short Answer/Fill-in-the-Blank

1 List the reasons why studying preparing for licensure and employment is important for a barber.

a. ____

____

____

____

b. ____

____

____

____

c. ____

____

____

____

2 No matter what changes occur in the economy, there are often more jobs available for ____________________ barbers than there are people to fill them.

3 You must thoroughly ____________________ the job market in your ____________________ area before committing to your first job.

Why Study Preparing for Licensure and Employment?

Multiple Choice

4 Barbers should have a thorough understanding of preparing for licensure and employment because:

a. They will be able to teach others in the future.

b. They will receive a refund in tuition upon passing the exam.

c. It will help them find and land the best job for them.

d. They will receive a refund in tuition upon finding employment.

Prepare for Licensure

LO 1 **Describe the process of taking and passing your state licensing examinations.**

Preparing for the Written Exam

Fill-in-the-Blank

5 Complete the following habits of test-wise students:

- Have a planned, realistic study ________________.
- ________________ content carefully and become an ________________ studier.
- Keep well-organized ________________.
- Develop a detailed ________________ list.
- Take effective notes during ________________.
- Organize and review ________________.
- Review past ________________ and ________________.
- Listen carefully in class for ________________ and ________________ about what could be expected on the test.

6 Avoid ________________ the night before an examination.

On Test Day

Multiple Choice

7 On test day, it is important to ______________________.

a. spend more than enough time on each question

b. slowly mark the answers on the test

c. relax and try to slow down physically

d. answer the difficult questions first

8 ______________________ before beginning.

a. Carefully read each question

b. Turn up your cell phone

c. Mark down *c* for every question

d. Scan the entire test

9 For questions that cause uncertainty, ______________________.

a. guess

b. leave blank

c. answer *c*

d. focus until you can be sure of your answer

Deductive Reasoning

Fill-in-the-Blank

10 Deductive reasoning is the process of reaching logical ______________________ by employing logical ______________________.

11 Complete the following deductive reasoning strategies:

- Eliminate options that are known to be ______________________.
- Watch for ______________________ or terms. Look for any ______________________ conditions or statements.
- Study the ______________________, which is the basic question or problem.
- When questions include paragraphs to read and questions to answer, read the ______________________ first.

Understanding Test Formats

Short Answer

12 The most important strategy of test taking is to know your material. Provide two additional tips for each question type below:

TRUE/FALSE

- ____
  ____
- ____
  ____

MULTIPLE CHOICE

- ______________________________
  ____
  ____
  ____
  ____
- ______________________________
  ____
  ____
  ____
  ____

MATCHING

- ______________________________
  ____
- ______________________________
  ____

ESSAYS

- ______________________________
  ____
- ______________________________
  ____

Barber Law

Fill-in-the-Blank

13 Complete the following barber law and regulation questions that may vary from state to state:

- Number of ______________ members.
- Terms of ______________.
- Examination ______________.
- ______________ display.
- License ______________ dates.
- ______________ education requirements.

The Practical Exam

True or False

14 For the following statements, circle T if true or F if false.

T **F** The basic skills or procedures that are usually evaluated are haircutting, shaving, shampooing, and possibly blowdrying or a chemical service.

T **F** Practice the correct skills required for the test as often as you can, preferably on a variety of hair types.

T **F** To be better prepared for the practical portion of the examination, participate in mock licensing examinations; complete with timed sections.

T **F** Make a list of equipment and implements that will be provided for you during the examination.

T **F** Make certain your appearance is neat, clean, and professional.

Prepare for Employment

LO 2 **Develop a resume and employment portfolio.**

How to Get the Job You Want, Where You Want

Matching/Fill-in-the-Blank

15 Match the correct personal characteristic with its description.

_____ The compass that keeps you on course over the long haul of your career

_____ The drive to take the necessary action to achieve a goal

_____ Must both be developed to reach the level of success you desire

_____ Taking pride in your work and committing yourself to consistently doing a good job

_____ Eagerness to learn, grow, and expand your skills and knowledge

a. Enthusiasm

b. Good technical and communication skills

c. Integrity

d. Motivation

e. Strong work ethic

16 While the vast majority of barbers do work in barbershops, some perform services in either _______________ or _______________ salons.

17 _______________ is possibly the least expensive way of owning your own business.

Resume Development

Short Answer/True or False

18 Give four basic guidelines to follow when preparing your professional resume.

- ______________________________
- ______________________________
- ______________________________
- ______________________________

19 How can you show concrete accomplishment on your resume?

____

20 What are three questions you should consider regarding your accomplishments during school?

- ______________________________
- ______________________________
- ______________________________

21 For the following dos and don'ts of resume writing, circle T if true or F if false.

T **F** Include all contact information

T **F** Make your resume hard to read

T **F** Keep your resume long

T **F** Stress accomplishments

T **F** Focus on hobbies

T **F** Emphasize transferable skills

T	**F**	Use passive verbs
T	**F**	Make your resume neat
T	**F**	Avoid professional references
T	**F**	State salary history
T	**F**	Include a cover letter
T	**F**	Do not include computer skills

Employment Portfolio

Mind Mapping/Short Answer

22 Create a mind map of elements you would include in your portfolio.

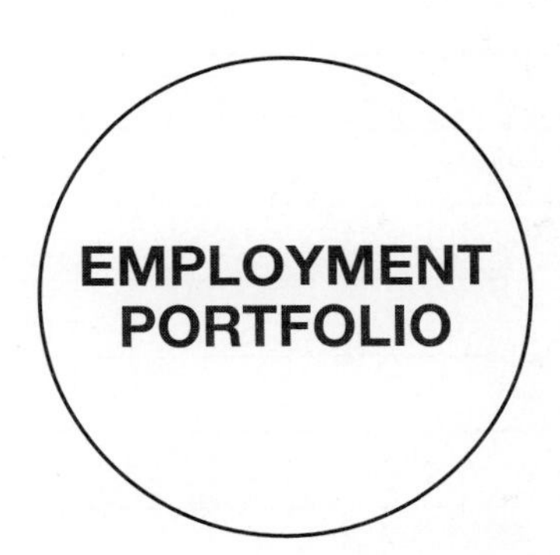

23 What are some ways that you can create an online or electronic portfolio of your work?

____

____

____

____

____

Targeting the Establishment, Field Research, and the Barbershop Visit

Case Study/Fill-in-the-Blank

24 Your Future Job

Barbering students are advised to explore the job market and research potential employers even before they graduate, not least because it takes time to get hired. Although students may take shortcuts, often at their own expense, there are steps to follow in finding a good job and getting hired. Explain the benefits of exploring the job market and researching potential employers. Also, describe the steps involved in finding a suitable establishment to work in and getting an interview there.

____

____

____

____

____

____

____

____

____

____

25 A great way to find out about potential jobs is to _______________.

26 When you visit the barbershop, take along a _______________ to ensure that you observe all the _______________ that might ultimately affect your decision making.

27 After your visit, always remember to _______________ with a handwritten _______________ or _______________, thanking the barbershop representative for his time.

Arrange for a Job Interview

LO 3 Know how to explore the job market, research potential employers, and operate within the legal aspects of employment.

Interview Preparation

Short Answer

28 List three specific components for each of the following necessary interview materials:

IDENTIFICATION

- ______________________________
- ______________________________
- ______________________________

INTERVIEW WARDROBE

- ______________________________
- ______________________________
- ______________________________

SUPPORTING MATERIALS

- ______________________________
- ______________________________
- ______________________________

29 What are three typical interview questions you should review and prepare for?

- ______________________________
- ______________________________
- ______________________________

The Interview

Fill-in-the-Blank

30 Complete the following behaviors to be followed with the interview itself:

- Always be on time or, better yet, ______________________.
- Turn ______________________ your cell phone.
- Project a warm, friendly ______________________ . ______________________ is the universal language.
- Do not come to an interview with anything to ______________________ or ______________________ .
- Do not ______________________ before you are ready, and not for more than ______________________ at a time.
- Never ______________________ former employers.
- Always remember to ______________________ the interviewer at the end of the interview.

31 Come to an interview prepared to ask questions, but do not feel that you have to ask all of them. The point is to create as much of a ______________________ as possible.

32 Close the interview with ______________________ that you want the job (if you do).

Legal Aspects of the Employment Interview and Employee Contracts

Short Answer

33 Write permissible questions to ask during an interview regarding the following topics:

Age or date of birth

____

____

Disabilities or physical traits

____

____

Citizenship

____

____

Language fluency

____

____

34 What are noncompete agreements?

____

____

____

____

The Employment Application and Doing It Right

Fill-in-the-Blank

35 Any time that you are applying for any position, you will be required to complete an ______________________, even if your ______________________ already contains much of the requested information.

36 Once you are employed, be sure to read all you can about the ______________________, attend ______________________, and take advantage of as much ______________________ as you can manage.

Word Review

Short Answer

Fill in the definition for the following terms.

Deductive reasoning

____

____

Employment portfolio

____

____

Practical exam

____

____

Resume

____

____

Stem

____

____

Test-wise

____

____

Transferable skills

____

____

Work ethic

____

____

CHAPTER 20 WORKING BEHIND THE CHAIR

LEARNING OBJECTIVES

After completing this chapter, you will be able to:

LO1 **Describe what is expected of a new employee and what this means in terms of your everyday behavior.**

LO2 **List the habits of a good barbershop team player.**

LO3 **Describe three different ways in which barbers are compensated.**

LO4 **Determine the best way to record your tips and make additional income.**

LO5 **Explain the principles of selling products and services in the barbershop.**

LO6 **List the most effective ways to build a client base.**

Introduction

Short Answer/Fill-in-the-Blank

1 List two reasons why studying working behind the chair is important for a barber.

a. ____

____

____

b. ____

____

____

2 It is important to prioritize your ____________________ and commit to personal ____________________ of conduct and behavior.

Why Study Working Behind the Chair?

Multiple Choice

3 Barbers should have a thorough understanding of working behind the chair because:

a. Barbers will be tested on the topic during their evaluation.

b. It will help barbers belong to and work as a team.

c. The knowledge can be shared with clients.

d. It will help keep clients safe.

Describe the Expectations of Moving from School to Work

LO 1 **Describe what is expected of a new employee and what this means in terms of your everyday behavior.**

True/False

4 For the following statements, circle T if true or F if false.

T **F** Barbering school is an unforgiving environment.

T **F** When you work in a barbershop, you will be expected to put the needs of the barbershop and its clients ahead of your own.

T **F** If someone comes to you with tickets for a concert on a day when you are scheduled to work, you should call your manager to take the day off.

Understanding the Real World

LO 2 **List the habits of a good barbershop team player.**

LO 3 **Describe three different ways in which barbers are compensated.**

Thriving in a Service Profession and Barbershop Teamwork

Short Answer

5 List the guidelines for meeting your clients' needs in a service position.

- ____________________
- ____________________
- ____________________
- ____________________
- ____________________

6 Give four workplace principles you should practice to become a good team player.

- ____________________
- ____________________
- ____________________
- ____________________
- ____________________
- ____________________
- ____________________
- ____________________

The Job Description

Fill-in-the-Blank

7 A job description is a document that ____________________ all the ____________________ and ____________________ of a particular position in a barbershop.

8 If you find yourself at a shop that does not use job descriptions, you may want to ______________________.

9 The best job descriptions outline not only the employee's duties and responsibilities, but also the ______________________ expected of them and the ______________________ available to them.

Employment Classifications

Matching

10 Match the correct employment status with each description.

_____ Should receive a Form 1099-MISC from the shop owner

_____ Handles all money transactions

_____ Works on a salary, commission, or salary-plus-commission basis

_____ May be (and needs to be) renewed periodically

_____ Wholly responsible for clientele, supplies, record keeping, maintenance, and accounting

_____ Status of the fewest barbers

_____ Leases space from the shop owner

_____ Rents a chair or works for a percentage of performed service proceeds

_____ Likely doesn't handle money, beyond tips

_____ Is set up as a small business

_____ Is not responsible for withholding income and Medicare taxes

a. Employee

b. Independent contractor

c. Booth renter

Wage Structures

Multiple Choice/Fill-in-the-Blank

11 An example of the ______________________ wage structure is receiving 60% of the $400 in gross sales you generated.

a. salary

b. commission

c. salary-plus-commission

d. tip

12 An example of the ______________________ wage structure is receiving $15 per hour worked and 40% of the $400 in gross sales you generated.

a. salary

b. commission

c. salary-plus-commission

d. tip

13 An example of the ______________ wage structure is receiving $17 per hour worked and 0% of the $200 in gross sales you generated.

a. salary
b. commission
c. salary-plus-commission
d. tip

14 A salary-plus-commission is sometimes called a ______________.

15 ______________ are income in addition to your regular compensation and must be tracked and reported on your income tax return.

16 With ______________, all the fees brought in from the performance of services are basically yours after paying for the rent and supplies.

Employee Evaluation

Short Answer

17 Who are three people you might approach to evaluate your work and provide feedback?

- ______________________________
- ______________________________
- ______________________________

18 How can you find and get help from a role model?

____

____

____

____

____

____

____

____

____

____

Manage Your Money

LO 4 **Determine the best way to record your tips and make additional income.**

Repaying Your Debts and Reporting Your Income

Fill-in-the-Blank/Case Study

19 Not paying back your loans is called ______________, and it can have serious consequences regarding your personal and professional ______________.

20 Before committing to a ________________________, make sure you understand the payment ________________________, interest ________________________, and what you realistically can ________________________.

21 When you complete your yearly taxes, it is critical that you report ________________________ and ________________________ that is not shown on your paycheck.

22 The best way to record your tips and additional income is to keep a ________________________.

23 As you begin to think about going on a budget, ask yourself: What is your ________________________ after all your ________________________ are paid?

24 Make More Money

Barbers are paid in a number of ways, including a salary, commission, or both, as well as tips. However, there may come a time when additional income is needed. If you were paid a salary that does not take overtime into account and received 35% commission on gross sales you make, how would you go about earning additional income?

____

____

____

____

____

____

____

____

Discover the Selling You

LO 5 Explain the principles of selling products and services in the barbershop.

Fill-in-the-Blank

25 ________________________, also known as *upselling*, is the practice of recommending and selling additional ________________________ to your clients.

26 ________________________ is the act of recommending and selling ________________________ to your clients for at-home use.

The Principles and Psychology of Selling

Short Answer

27 List four principles of selling barbering products and services.

-
-
-
-

28 Give four tips on how to get the conversation started on retailing products.

-
-
-
-

29 What are the five points to keep in mind when selling?

1.
2.
3.
4.
5.

Keep Current Clients and Expand Your Client Base

LO 6 **List the most effective ways to build a client base.**

Short Answer

30 Explain why it may be a good idea to ask for and record a client's birth date (just the month and day, not the year).

31 Explain how social media can be used to build your reputation and attract new clients.

32 Explain how a business card referral system can be used to build clientele.

Rebooking Clients

Fill-in-the-Blank

33 The best time to think about getting your clients back into the shop is ______________________.

34 Listen carefully to what your clients tell you ______________________ their visit, because they will often give ______________________ as to what is happening in their lives.

On Your Way

Fill-in-the-Blank

35 Your first job in this industry will most likely be the most ______________________.

36 Make use of the many generous and experienced ______________________ you will encounter.

37 Above all, always be willing to ______________________.

Word Review

Word Scramble

Unscramble the key term, using the provided definitions as clues.

obtoh nlater ____

Also known as chair rental; a form of self-employment, business ownership, and tax designation, distinguished by renting a booth or station in a barbershop.

teincl easb ____

Customers who are loyal to a particular cosmetologist.

oissimmcn ____

A percentage of the revenue that the barbershop takes in from services performed by an employee, usually offered to that employee once the individual has built up a loyal clientele.

eeyploem ____

Employment classification in which the employer withholds certain taxes and has a high level of control.

netnedlpden otactrrnoc ____

A form of self-employment and tax designation with specific responsibilities for bookkeeping, taxes, insurances, and so on.

oJb oiptnricsed ______________________________

Document that outlines all the duties and responsibilities of a particular position in a barbershop or spa.

ingrateli ______________________________

The act of recommending and selling products to your clients for at-home use.

ktetci dangigpru ______________________________

Also known as upselling services; the practice of recommending and selling additional services to your clients.

LEARNING OBJECTIVES

After completing this chapter, you will be able to:

LO1 **Identify two options for going into business for yourself.**

LO2 **List the basic factors to be considered when opening a barbershop.**

LO3 **Compare types of barbershop ownership.**

LO4 **Recognize the information that should be included in a business plan.**

LO5 **Explain the importance of record keeping.**

LO6 **Examine the responsibilities of a booth renter.**

LO7 **Distinguish the elements of successful barbershop operations.**

LO8 **Validate why advertising is a vital aspect of a barbershop's success.**

Introduction

Short Answer

1 List two reasons why studying the business of barbering is important for a barber.

a. ______________________________

____

____

b. ______________________________

____

____

Why Study the Business of Barbering?

Multiple Choice

2 Barbers should have a thorough understanding of the business of barbering because:

a. It will help you manage your career.

b. It will help you start a career in teaching barbering.

c. It is a requirement of state barber boards.

d. Clients would prefer them to cut their hair over other barbers.

Review Types of Business Options

LO 1 **Identify two options for going into business for yourself.**

LO 2 **List the basic factors to be considered when opening a barbershop.**

LO 3 **Compare types of barbershop ownership.**

LO 4 **Recognize the information that should be included in a business plan.**

LO 5 **Explain the importance of record keeping.**

Fill-in-the-Blank

3 If you want to become your own boss, you have two main options to consider: (1) ____________________ or (2) ______________________________.

4 Both options require significant ____________________ investment and a strong line of ____________________, and there is no guarantee of ____________________.

Opening Your Own Barbershop

Short Answer/Matching

5 List four general decisions that must be made before opening a shop.

- ______________________________
- ______________________________
- ______________________________
- ______________________________

6 Identify three questions that should be answered when creating a brand identity.

- ______________________________
- ______________________________
- ______________________________

7 What is a mission statement and what does it do?

____

____

____

____

____

8 Fill in the year ranges to complete the business timeline below. The first has been done for you.

Year 1	Time spent determining and completing all aspects of starting the business.
______________	Time period for tending to the business, its clientele, and its employees and for growing and expanding.
______________	Time period for adding more locations, expanding the scope of the business, constructing a larger space, etc.
______________	Time to consider moving from being a working barber to a full-time manager of the business and planning for eventual retirement.
______________	Time to consider selling the business or training a junior partner to take over day-to-day operations.

9 Match the terms below with their descriptions.

_____ Any and all local, state, and federal regulations and laws that must be complied with

_____ Explains what a business is and identifies characteristics that set it apart from competitors

_____ Act of maintaining accurate and complete records of all financial activities

_____ Ideally has good visibility, high traffic, easy access, sufficient parking, and handicap access

_____ Whether certain practical issues of a business have been addressed or not

_____ Documents that detail, usually for legal purposes, who does what and what is given in return

_____ Written description of the business today and in the next 5 years (detailed by year)

_____ Ongoing, recurring processes or activities involved in running a barbershop for income and value

_____ Information about a specific population, including data on race, age, income, education, etc.

_____ Rules and regulations adopted by a barbershop to ensure that all clients and associates are treated fairly and consistently

_____ Guarantees protection against financial loss from malpractice, property liability, fire, burglary and theft, and business interruption

a. Barbershop operation

b. Barbershop policies

c. Business feasibility

d. Business name

e. Business plan

f. Business regulations and laws

g. Demographics

h. Insurance

i. Location

j. Written agreements

k. Record keeping

Types of Barbershop Ownership

Matching/True or False

10 Match the correct company structure with each description.

_____ Raises capital by issuing stock certificates or shares

_____ Two or more people assume one another's liability for debts

_____ Requires paying a fee to a firm that is already successful, regardless of profit

_____ Individual owner assumes expenses, receives profits, and bears all losses

_____ Trust is just one of the requirements

_____ Individual owner determines policies and has the last say in decision making

_____ Offers protection of personal assets

_____ Offers the advantage of a known name and brand recognition

a. Sole proprietorship

b. Partnership

c. Corporation

d. Franchise

11 For the following statements, circle T if true or F if false.

T **F** With a corporation, income tax is limited to the salary that you draw and not the total profits of the business.

T **F** One reason for going into a partnership arrangement is to have more capital, or money to invest in a business; another is to have help running your operation.

T **F** If you like to make your own rules and are responsible enough to meet all the duties and obligations of running a business, a franchise may be the best arrangement for you.

Business Plan

Word Search

12 Find the information and materials that should be included in a business plan in the word search and list them in the blanks below.

1. ______________________
2. ______________________
3. ______________________
4. ______________________
5. ______________________
6. ______________________
7. ______________________
8. ______________________

E	E	B	S	N	M	P	N	O	O	C	N	T	N	E	R	G	N	O
X	M	A	R	K	E	T	I	N	G	P	L	A	N	L	N	S	B	A
E	F	R	P	R	S	O	D	N	T	N	T	T	E	P	A	S	R	P
C	O	B	R	L	S	V	N	S	P	T	M	T	I	A	P	U	T	N
U	O	E	C	E	I	S	S	A	N	T	T	P	S	P	E	M	S	S
T	O	R	G	A	N	I	Z	A	T	I	O	N	A	L	P	L	A	N
I	O	S	E	S	N	I	B	O	C	S	M	E	S	E	A	E	P	C
V	V	H	A	K	O	I	U	A	T	L	I	P	R	N	T	N	I	C
E	L	O	A	E	A	U	E	B	N	A	P	M	N	R	T	E	V	R
S	U	P	P	O	R	T	I	N	G	D	O	C	U	M	E	N	T	S
U	E	P	N	N	I	I	A	A	N	T	O	E	A	A	T	D	H	M
M	N	O	I	K	N	P	I	O	T	N	C	E	I	P	T	C	E	I
M	O	L	E	P	P	T	S	T	O	N	I	S	L	T	I	O	M	O
A	V	I	S	I	O	N	S	T	A	T	E	M	E	N	T	M	C	T
R	I	C	I	K	C	C	R	N	C	V	C	S	Y	M	M	E	T	O
Y	F	I	N	A	N	C	I	A	L	D	O	C	U	M	E	N	T	S
T	R	E	M	M	N	N	N	E	A	P	G	P	L	O	S	A	S	N
M	I	S	S	I	O	N	S	T	A	T	E	M	E	N	T	E	I	T
G	O	E	L	U	E	S	L	O	N	E	O	G	P	E	L	A	A	E

Purchasing an Established Barbershop and Drawing Up a Lease

Fill-in-the-Blank

13 Complete the following items that should be included in any agreement to buy an established barbershop:

- A ________________ to determine the ________________ value of the business once the current owner's ________________ are taken out of the equation.
- Use of the barbershop's ________________ and ________________ for a ________________ period of time.
- Disclosure of the ________________ of the facility, including a full ________________ if you are buying the actual ________________.
- ________________ agreement stating that the seller will not work in or establish ________________ within ________________ from the present location.
- An ________________ agreement that lets you know if the ________________ will stay with the business under its new ownership. Existing contracts should be ________________.

14 Complete the following items you should secure when drawing up a lease:

- Exemption of ________________ or ________________ that might be attached to the barbershop so that they can be ________________.
- Agreement about necessary ________________ and ________________.
- Option from the landlord that allows you to assign the ________________ to ________________.

Protection Against Fire, Theft, and Lawsuits

Short Answer

15 Give three ways in which you can reduce risk and ensure the protection of your business, clients, and staff.

1. ____

____

____

2. ____

____

____

3. ____

____

____

Business Operations and the Importance of Record Keeping

Short Answer/Case Study

16 What two things do you need to run a people-oriented business?

1. ______________________________

2. ______________________________

17 Smooth business management depends on what factors?

____

____

____

____

____

18 Good Record Keeping

Proper business records are necessary to meet the requirements of local, state, and federal laws regarding taxes and employees. They also help to keep the business operating efficiently. Failure to keep good records can cause the business to suffer. Explain the consequences of not keeping good product and service records, purchase and inventory records, and expense records.

____

____

____

____

____

____

____

____

Understand Booth Rental

LO 6 **Examine the responsibilities of a booth renter.**

Fill-in-the-Blank

19 Complete the following obligations of a booth renter.

- Keeping ____________ for ____________ purposes and other legal reasons.
- Paying all ____________, including higher Social Security ____________ that of an employee.
- Carrying adequate ____________ insurance and ____________ insurance.

- Complying with all IRS obligations for ______________________.
- Using your own ______________________ and ______________________ systems.
- Collecting all ______________________ fees, whether they are paid in ______________________ or via ______________________.
- Creating all ______________________ materials, including business cards and a service menu.
- Purchasing of all ______________________, including ______________________ and ______________________ supplies and products.
- ______________________ and ______________________ inventory.
- Budgeting for ______________________ or offering ______________________ to ensure a steady flow of new clients.
- Pay for all continuing ______________________.
- Adhering to state ______________________ and ______________________. To date, two states ______________________ and ______________________ do not allow booth rental at all.

Understand the Elements of a Successful Barbershop

LO 7 **Distinguish the elements of successful barbershop operations.**

Planning the Barbershop's Layout

Multiple Choice

20 ____________________ should be the primary concern when it comes to a barbershop's layout.

a. Maximum efficiency
b. Refreshments
c. Retail space
d. Good conversation

21 If you are opening a high-end barbershop, you may want to plan for more room in the ____________________.

a. storage room
b. break room
c. restrooms
d. waiting area

22 Costs to create even a small barbershop in an existing space can range from ____________________ per square foot.

a. \$25 to \$50
b. \$50 to 75
c. \$75 to \$125
d. \$125 to \$200

23 It takes most new shops about ____________________ to begin operating at full capacity.

a. 1 month
b. 6 months
c. 1 year
d. 2 to 5 years

Personnel

Short Answer

24 List the factors to consider when interviewing potential employees.

- ____________________
- ____________________
- ____________________
- ____________________
- ____________________
- ____________________

25 Explain how to can give your staff incentives.

____

____

____

____

____

26 What are two civil rights laws that employers must be familiar with?

- ____________________
- ____________________

The Front Desk

Fill-in-the-Blank

27 First impressions count, and since the ____________ area is the first area clients see, it needs to be attractive, ____________, and ____________.

28 The ____________ should have an ____________ that reflects your ____________, should be pleasant and ____________, should greet each client with a ____________, and should ____________ each client by name.

29 The receptionist should have a thorough knowledge of all ____________ carried by the shop so that they can also serve as ____________ and ____________ source for clients.

30 The key duty of the receptionist is ____________.

31 Appointments must be scheduled to make the most ____________ use of everyone's time—both the ____________ and the ____________.

32 Anyone who ____________ or deals with clients must have a pleasing ____________ and ____________.

Use of Telephone in the Barbershop

Fill-in-the-Blank

33 When using the telephone, you should show ________________ and ________________ when talking with a client or ________________.

34 Answer the phone ________________. A good rule of thumb is to not let the phone ring more than ________________ times.

35 When booking appointments, take down the client's first and last ________________, their phone ________________, their ________________ address, and the ________________ booked.

36 When handling a complaint by phone, respond with ________________, ________________, and ________________, no matter how trying the circumstances.

Know How to Build Your Business

LO 8 **Validate why advertising is a vital aspect of a barbershop's success.**

Social Media

Short Answer

37 List some guidelines to effectively using social media.

- ____
- ____
- ____
- ____

Advertising

True or False/Short Answer

38 For the following statements, circle T if true or F if false.

T **F** The first goal of every business should be to maintain current clients.

T **F** Satisfied clients are the worst form of advertising.

T **F** By having a prebooking system in place, you are guaranteeing that you won't have repeat business.

39 Give the advertising tools you may choose to attract customers to your barbershop.

1. ____________________
2. ____________________
3. ____________________
4. ____________________
5. ____________________
6. ____________________
7. ____________________
8. ____________________
9. ____________________
10. ____________________
11. ____________________
12. ____________________
13. ____________________
14. ____________________

Selling in the Barbershop

Multiple Choice

40 ____________________ is the selling of take-home or maintenance products.

a. Upselling
b. Retailing
c. Cross promoting
d. Downselling

41 An example of ____________________ is encouraging a client who is booked for a haircut to also get a facial.

a. upselling
b. retailing
c. cross promoting
d. downselling

42 ____________________ is the adding on of additional services.

a. Upselling
b. Retailing
c. Cross promoting
d. Downselling

Word Review

Short Answer

Fill in the definition for the following terms.

Barbershop operation

Capital

Demographics

Goals

Insurance

Partnership

Record keeping

Social media

Vision statement

Written agreement